PANCREATIC ISLET
CELL REGENERATION
AND GROWTH

ADVANCES IN EXPERIMENTAL MEDICINE AND BIOLOGY

Recent Volumes in this Series

PANCREATIC ISLET CELL REGENERATION AND GROWTH

Edited by

Aaron I. Vinik

The Diabetes Institutes
Eastern Virginia Medical School
Norfolk, Virginia

Associate Editor:

Etta J. Vinik

Assistant Editor:

David J. Sirman

SPRINGER SCIENCE+BUSINESS MEDIA, LLC

Library of Congress Cataloging in Publication Data

Pancreatic islet cell regeneration and growth / edited by Aaron I. Vinik: associate
editor, Etta J. Vinik: assistant editor, David J. Sirman.
     p.   cm. — (Advances in experimental medicine and biology; v. 321)
   "Proceedings of the Diabetes Institute Conference on Islet Cell Regeneration and
Growth, held June 22-23, 1991, in Norfolk, Virginia" — T.p. verso.
   Includes bibliographical references and index.
   ISBN 978-0-306-44259-9   ISBN 978-1-4615-3448-8 (eBook)
   DOI 10.1007/978-1-4615-3448-8
   1. Islands of Langerhans — Regeneration — Congresses. 2. Islands of Langerhans —
Growth — Congresses. I. Vinik, Aaron I. II. Vinik, Etta J. III. Sirman, David J. IV.
Diabetes Institute Conference on Islet Cell Regeneration and Growth (1991: Norfolk,
Va.) V. Series.
   [DNLM: 1. Growth Substances. 2. Islets of Langerhans — growth & development. 3.
Islets of Langerhans — physiology. 4. Regeneration — genetics. W1 AD559 v. 321 / WI
802 P188]
QP188.P26P36 1992
612.3'4 — dc20
DNLM/DLC   92-49923
for Library of Congress   CIP

ISBN 978-0-306-44259-9

Proceedings of the Diabetes Institute Conference on Islet Cell
Regeneration and Growth, held June 22-23, 1991, in Norfolk, Virginia

© 1992 Springer Science+Business Media New York
Originally published by Plenum Press, New York in 1992

ACKNOWLEDGEMENTS

The success of the symposium on islet growth and differentiation and the timely publication of this volume were made possible by the contributions of a number of people and organizations. Special thanks are due to Leon-Paul Georges, M.D., Director of the Diabetes Institutes at Eastern Virginia Medical School for his enthusiasm and generous support that made the symposium and its accompanying social activities possible. Thanks are also due to the Diabetes Foundation whose raison d'etre is supporting our efforts to find the cure for diabetes and its complications, and in so doing, this symposium.

I would like to thank Etta Vinik, the associate director of the Education Institute for arranging a meeting of participants and visitors from near and far who were able to interact in a milieu conducive to intense periods of information exchange accompanied by congeniality and the spirit of comeraderie so essential to forging future relationships. Etta is to be thanked for her considerable effort in goading the participants to submit their contributions in a timely manner, thereafter proofreading the manuscripts for consistency, grammar, and typographical errors. David Sirman has heroically attended to the details of presentation and systematically reformatted each submission so that there is an appearance of uniformity throughout. Plenum Press are to be thanked for publishing this volume and for their cooperation in bringing the project to its natural conclusion. Lastly, I extend my sincere thanks to all the contributors to this volume for the outstanding quality of their chapters and their prompt responses which made the publication a timely one.

Aaron I. Vinik, M.D., Ph.D.

CONTENTS

SECTION THREE - INDUCTION OF CELL GROWTH AND MECHANISMS

SECTION FOUR - PATHOGENIC AND THERAPEUTIC RAMIFICATIONS

INTRODUCTION

Aaron I. Vinik, M.D., Ph.D.[1]

[1]Eastern Virginia Medical School
The Diabetes Institutes
Norfolk, Virginia 23510

This symposium, held in June 1991, was a gathering of international scientists to exchange their views on current concepts of cell growth and differentiation. Each scientist was asked to present a topic of their research related to cell growth and regeneration and to participate in a round table conference elaborating on current knowledge and sharing their experiences. By furthering this promising area of endeavor, a means of understanding ontogeny of cell development and of providing insights into tumor biology would prevail. Of prime importance was the anticipation that new information from a better understanding of the normal evolution of the pancreatic islet would generate alternative approaches to curing diabetes. This forward serves as a short introduction to the concept of pancreatic islet regeneration and the models currently in use to study the process.

DEVELOPMENTAL ORIGIN OF ISLETS DURING EMRYOGENESIS

The developing pancreas appears as a protrusion from the dorsal surface of the embryonic gut.[1] The different islet cell types appear sequentially during development *in vivo*. It therefore seems reasonable to propose that coordinated growth is dependent upon specificity of growth factors.

Islet cells *in vivo* also express several neuroectodermal antigens, for example, PGP 9.5,[2] neurone-specific enolase (NSE),[3] synaptophysin,[4] A2B5,[5] phenylethanolamine N-methyl-transferase (PNMT) and aromatic amino acid decarboxylase (AADC).[6] The endocrine cells of the GEP axis are capable of amine precursor uptake and decarboxylation and have, therefore, been given the acronym APUD.[7] The morphologic similarity of APUD cells suggested a common embryologic origin, which was believed to be the neural crest but later revised to include the neuroectoderm, or in the case of some of the endocrine cells, from the dorsal placoderm.

Studies by Ledouarin,[8] Pictet,[9] Andrew,[10] and their coworkers have cast doubt on this hypothesis, and most workers agree that these cells should be classified according to their secretory products, i.e., gastrin, somatostatin, glucagon. PP, etc. However, it is now thought that β–cells do not have APUD characteristics and are likely to be derived from gut, but express neuronal antigens such as the catecholamine biosynthetic enzyme tyrosine hydroxylase (TH).[11] The generally held belief that the neuronal characteristics of these cells indicated an ectodermal origin during mammalian embryogencsis has largely been dispelled.

During development *in vivo*, the phenotype of the mature islet cells appear sequentially. β-cells arise from progenitor cells localized in the pancreatic duct and these precursors transiently express TH while migrating away from the duct to populate a new islet. This suggests that the pancreatic duct is a source of endocrine stem cells throughout embryogenesis without the need to postulate a neuroendocrine origin. This notion is supported by the finding that the embryonic pancreatic duct *in vitro* is able to regenerate a new pancreas containing exocrine and endocrine cells expressing only peptides (mature cells), and cells containing both TH and a hormone (immature cells).[12,13]

Teitelman has shown that pancreatic cells of endocrine origin can indeed express several neuronal antigens in addition to the peptide hormones.[11] She further showed that in the mouse embryo a primitive undifferentiated cell(s) led to sequential appearance of at least 4 different cell types containing either a hormone (e.g., glucagon), a catecholamine enzyme (tyrosine hydroxylase, TH) or combinations of these.[6] Under appropriate conditions these cells can be shown to differentiate into either neurites or adult endocrine cells. During regeneration, expression of neural antigens by developing cells was found to constitute an early phase to be replaced by the adult hormone secreting counterpart. Rosenberg and Vinik[14] have utilized a model for nesidioblastosis and shown that pancreatic ductal cells are capable of differentiating upon stimulation into adult endocrine cells capable of secreting insulin in a fully regulated manner.

ISLET CELL GROWTH AND DIFFERENTIATION

Factors which control the growth and functional maturation and differentiation of the human endocrine pancreas and gut during the fetal and post-natal periods are incompletely understood. The role of the fetal mesenchyme in epithelial cell development and differentiation appears to be important.[15-17] Possible mechanisms of action include: (i) secretion of an inducing or transforming hormonal growth factor, (ii) information exchange through cell-to-cell contact via paracrine and juxtacrine actions of locally elaborated growth factors, and (iii) production of an extracellular matrix rich in growth promoting factors. The soluble peptide growth factors are trophic substances that regulate both cell proliferation and differentiation and may be linked to islet growth.

One family of growth factors that may be implicated in islet growth are the somatomedins and their binding proteins. Insulin-like growth factors (IGFs) are important mediators of fetal and postnatal growth. Whereas these growth factors circulate (attached to binding proteins) they also act locally. Fetal rat islets release both IGF-I and IGF-II *in vitro* which may contribute to growth hormone-induced DNA synthesis.[18-21] It is apparent that the role of IGF-I, and the binding proteins, especially in the adult pancreas is far from clear. In this symposium Drs. LeRoith and Lauterio discuss aspects of IGF physiology, and LeRoith focuses upon differences in the role of the IGF's in regeneration of adult and fetal tissues. Dr. Hill emphasizes the role of the IGF's and their binding proteins in islet regeneration in the fetal pancreas at a time when the pancreas is susceptible to the influence of this particular group of growth factors. Dr. Bonner Weir also points out that in their model of islet regeneration after 90% pancreatectomy there is enhanced IGF gene expression in the ductules and certain connective tissue cells in contrast with the normal expression in capillary endothelial cells suggesting that IGFs may participate in the regeneration process after pancreatectomy in the rat.[22] Dr. Nielsen, however, contests the suggestion that the IGF's are important as pancreatic trophic factors and based upon his observations growth hormone itelf may be pertinent, at least in pregnancy, a state in which islet hypertrophy is found.

Several important glycoprotein components of extracellular matrix - the "integrins"- have also been recognized as playing a role in cell growth and differentiation. For example, fibronectin, laminin and tenascin.[23,24] Dr. Le Beau elaborates upon the role the integrins may play in cell regeneration. The role of these factors in the maintenance and replacement of a functional islet cell mass in the adult pancreas remains to be determined.

ISLET CELL PROLIFERATION IN THE POST-NATAL PERIOD

Several models designed to induce exocrine and endocrine pancreatic regeneration have been developed. In the model developed by Bonner-Weir and colleagues,[22,25] there is regeneration of both exocrine and endocrine tissue following a 90% pancreatectomy in which the increase in β–cell mass occurs as a result of the replication of existing β-cells and not necessarily because of a process of new islet formation.[22] This group have reported increased IGF-I mRNA production by capillary endothelial cells and proliferating ductules which may contribute to both endocrine and exocrine pancreas regeneration, but the precise role of IGFs needs to be elucidated and the possibility that other growth factors participate has not been excluded.[22]

Terazono et al developed a model in which 90% pancreatectomized rats or mice are treated with either nicotinamide, (a poly ADP-ribose synthetase inhibitor), or aurothioglucose resulting in exocrine and endocrine cell regeneration, and the appearance of a substance termed *reg* protein.[26,27] The gene encoding this protein has been termed the *reg* gene.[28] Human *reg* mRNA has been detected predominantly in the pancreas, and at lower levels in gastric mucosa and in the kidney.[29] *Reg* gene protein has also been found to be expressed ectopically in colon and rectal tumors,[29] linking enhanced *reg* expression to the transformed, proliferative state, at least for some cell types. Current evidence suggests that *reg* is expressed in acinar tissue and not regenerating islets. It may therefore be a paracrine growth factor. Dr. Okamoto, who pioneered the work on Reg gene and pancreatic regeneration, elaborates here upon his new findings. The controversy over the relevance of this growth factor in islet regeneration in other models is further discussed by Drs. Newgard and Rafaeloff.

Expression of an homologous gene, termed *rig*, has been identified in insulinoma tissue.[30] The significance of these genes remains to be determined. In both models of regeneration studied by Okamoto and colleagues,[26,27,29] islet size increased above normal over a period of weeks to months.

A second version of the 90% pancreatectomized rat model studied by Newgard and colleagues,[31] deals with *reg* expression in insulinoma-bearing New England Deaconess Hospital (NEDH) rats relative to normal controls and following tumor resection. They demonstrate that tumor implantation causes a sharp reduction in *reg* expression associated with a profound reduction in non-tumor islet size and that removal of the tumor, a maneuver that results in rapid β-cell proliferation, results in a large but transient induction in *reg* mRNA levels. Whether *reg* protein is β-cytotrophic is still an open question. The fact that high levels of *reg* mRNA are present in normal animals, in which β-cell replication is ongoing at a low, constitutive rate, are seemingly at odds with a growth-promoting role for this gene product.

Another model has been suggested by Dr. Sarvetnick[32] in which a regenerative process is observed in transgenic mice expressing Interferon-gamma in their pancreatic β-cells. These mice, in which diabetes ensues following immunodestruction of their β-cells, show duct cell proliferation and the appearance of more primitive neuroendocrine progenitor cells along the apical regions of the ducts. Dr. Sarvetnick discusses her most recent findings indicating that diabetes may not develop provided that the regenerative process outstrips the destructive process. This, we believe, is an important principle whereby an approach to induce regeneration may not be unreasonable in our quest for a cure for diabetes.

In 1982, we developed a unique model for islet regeneration in hamsters.[33,34] Hamsters 8 weeks of age are fertile, considered to be adult animals and respond better to the induction of cell proliferation than do older animals.[33,34] By producing partial obstruction of the hamster pancreatic duct by cellophane wrapping, new islet formation from ductal elements was observed. The mechanism by which partial obstruction in our model induces cell proliferation and differentiation is unknown. Using a parabiotic experimental design, these processes were shown to be mediated by paracrine and/or autocrine mechanisms.[30] Indeed, an extract prepared from a wrapped pancreas exhibited trophic activity when injected into other hamsters, but this was not observed when an extract prepared from a non-wrapped pancreas was administered. Drs. Rosenberg and Vinik review the data and the more recent developments in the use of a cytosol extract, containing the growth factor which we have called Ilotropin.

The presence of this specific growth factor, Ilotropin, in the β-cell cytosol extract has been hypothesized but the identity of the peptide had not been established. Dr. Pittenger reviews the current knowledge of the nature of the growth factor and the studies he has carried out to further define its characteristics. However, cellophane wrapping may initiate the release of a variety of growth factors that contribute to the coordinated, timely growth and differentiation of ductal cells. These possibilities and other factors that may be shared with factors important in the nervous system are highlighted by members of the faculty. The possible mechanism of action of the various factors as well as therapeutic applications are also discussed.

GROWTH FACTOR(S) AND NEOPLASIA

A great deal of interest is now being focused upon the factors responsible for initiation of growth, increase in cell number and size, differentiation into adult endocrine cells, growth cessation and cell maintenance.[36,37] The coincidental findings that the multiple endocrine neoplasia, type 1 syndrome (MEN-1) (combined occurrence of tumors of the pituitary, pancreas and parathyroid glands) is associated with the loss of alleles on chromosome 11,[38,39] the same chromosome on which the insulin gene has been located;[40] the finding of parathyroid mitogenic activity in the plasma of patients with MEN-1;[36,37] and evidence that patients with MEN-1 might also secrete mitogenic factors for pancreatic islet-cells into plasma,[41] suggests a role for genetically determined circulating growth factors in the 'growth initiation' of these tumors.

It is apparent, therefore, that the conference was timeous and that the information pertinent to our appreciation of cell growth and differentiation is relevant to a possible cure for diabetes as well as a clearer understanding of factors that may be involved in pancreatic tumor formation. Conceptually, these conditions represent the two ends of a spectrum - diabetes with endocrine cell failure and endocrine neoplasia with unbridled cell growth.

REFERENCES

1. R.L. Pictet and J.W. Rutter, Development of the embryonic endocrine pancreas, in: "Handbook of Physiology," D.F. Steiner and M. Frenkel, eds., Washington D.C., American Physiological Society (1972).
2. K.J. Thompson, J.F. Doran, P. Jackson, A.P. Dhillon, and J. Rode, PGP 9.5: a new marker for vertebrate neurons and endocrine cells, Brain Res. 278:224-28 (1983).
3. Polak, et al. Neuron-specific enolase, a marker for neuro-endocrine cells, in: Evolution and Tumor Pathology of the Neuro-endocrine System. Elsevier, New York (1984).
4. B. Weidenmann, W.W. Franke, C. Kuhn, R. Moll, and V.E. Gould, Synaptophysin: a marker protein for neuro-endocrine cells and neoplasms, Proc Natl Acad Sci USA. 83:3500-04 (1986).
5. G.S. Eisenbarth, K. Shimizu, M.A. Bowring, and S. Wells, Expression of receptors for fetanus toxin and monoclonal antibody A_2B_2 by pancreatic islet cells, Proc Natl Acad Sci USA. 79:5066-70 (1982).
6. G. Teitelman, T.H. Joh, and D.J. Reis, Transformation of catecholaminergic precursor into glucagon (A) cells in mouse embryonic pancreas, Proc Natl Acad Sci USA. 78:5225-29 (1991).
7. A.G.E. Pearse, Common cytochemical and ultrastructural characteristics of cells producing polypeptide hormones (the APUD series) and their relevance to thyroid and ultimobronchial C cells and calcitonin, Proc R Soc Lond (Biol). 170:71 (1968).
8. N.M. LeDouarian and M.A. Teillet, The migration of neural crest cells to the wall of the digestive tract in avian embryo, J Embryol Exp Morphol. 30:31 (1973).
9. R.L. Pictet, L.B. Rall, P. Phelps, and W.J. Rutter, The neural crest and the origin of the insulin-producing and other gastrointestinal hormone-producing cells, Science. 191:191 (1967).
10. A. Andrew, An experimental investigation into the possible neural crest origin of pancreatic APUD (islet) cells, J Embryol Exp Morphol. 35:577 (1976).
11. G. Teitelman and J.K. Lee, Cell lineage analysis of pancreatic islet cell development: Glucagon and insulin cells arise from catecholaminergic precursor present in the pancreatic duct, Devel Biol. 121:454-56 (1987).
12. G. Teitelman, J. Lee, and D.J. Reis, Differentiation of prospective mouse pancreatic islet cells during development in vitro and during regeneration, Dev Biol. 120:425-33 (1987).
13. R.W. Dudek and I.E. Lawrence, Morphologic evidence of interaction between adult ductal epithelium of pancreas and fetal foregut mesenchyme, Diabetes. 37:891-900 (1988).
14. L. Rosenberg, W.P. Duguid, and A.I. Vinik, Cell proliferation in the pancreas of the Syrian golden hamster, Dig Dis Sci. 32:1185 (1987).
15. R.L. Pictet, L. Rail, M. de Gasparo, and W.J. Rutter, Regulation of differentiation of endocrine cells during pancreatic development in-vitro, in: "Early diabetes in early life," R.A. Camerini-Davalos and H.S. Cole, eds., Academic Press, New York (1975).
16. B.S. Spooner, H.I. Cohen, and J. Faubion, Development of the embryonic mammalian pancreas: The relationship between morphogenesis and cytodifferentiation, Dev Biol. 61:119 (1977).
17. R. Montesano, P. Mouron, M. Amherdt, and L. Orci, Collagen matrix promotes reorganization of pancreatic endocrine cell monolayers into islet-like organoids, J Cell Biol. 97:935 (1983).
18. I. Sweene and D.J. Hill, Growth hormone regulation of DNA replication, but not insulin production, is partly mediated by somatomedin C/insulin-like growth factor-I in isolated pancreatic islets from adult rats, Diabetologia. 32:191-97 (1989).
19. D.J. Hill, A. Frazer, I. Swe, P.K. Wirdnam, and R.D.G. Milner, Somatostatin-C in human fetal pancreas, Diabetes. 36:465 (1987).

20. A. Rabinovitch, C. Quigley, T. Russell, Y. Patel, and D.H. Mintz, Insulin and multiplication stimulating activity (an insulin-like growth factor) stimulate islet β-cell replication in neonatal rat pancreatic monolayer cultures, Diabetes. 31:160 (1982).

21. J.M. Bryson, B.E. Tuch, and R.C. Baxter, Production of insulin-like growth factor-II by human fetal pancreas in culture, J Endocrinol. 121:367-73 (1989).

22. J.S. Brockenbrough, G.C. Weir, and S. Bonner-Weir, Discordance of exocrine and endocrine growth after 90% pancreatectomy in rats, Diabetes. 37:232-36 (1988).

23. M.J. Politis, Exogeneous laminin induces regenerative changes in traumatized sciatic and optic nerve, Plas Reconstr Surg. 83:228-35 (1989).

24. R. Chiquet-Ehrismann, E.J. Mackie, C.A. Pearson, and T. Sakakura, Tenascin: an extracellular matrix protein involved in tissue interactions during fetal development and oncogenesis, Cell. 47:131-39 (1986).

25. F. Smith, K. Rosen, L. Villa-Kamoroff, et al, Enhanced IGG-I gene expression in regenerating rat pancreas is localized to capillaries and proliferating ductules, Diabetes. 39(Suppl 1):66A (1990).

26. K. Terazono, H. Yamamoto, S. Takasawa, K. Shiga, Y. Yonemura, Y. Tochino, and H. Okamoto, A novel gene activated in regenerating islets, J Biol Chem. 262:2111 (1988).

27. K. Terazono, Y. Uchiyama, M. Ide, T. Watanabe, H. Yonekura, H. Yamamoto, and H. Okamoto, Expression of *reg* protein in rat regenerating islets and its co-localization with insulin in beta cell secretory granules, Diabetologia. 33:1 (1990).

28. T. Watanabe, H. Yonekura, K. Terazono, H. Yamamoto, and H. Okamoto, Complete nucleotide sequence of human *reg* gene and its expression in normal and tumoral tissues, J Biol Chem. 265:7432-39 (1990).

29. C. Miyaura, et al, Expression of *reg*/PSP, a pancreatic exocrine gene: Relationship to changes in islet β-cell mass, Mol Endocrinol. (1991, in press).

30. S. Takasawa, K. Yamamoto, K. Terazono, and H. Okamoto, Novel gene activated in rat insulinoma, Diabetes. 35:1178 (1986).

31. L. Chen, M. Appel, T. Alam, C. Miyaura, A. Sestak, J. O'Neil, R. Unger, and C. Newgard, Factors Regulating Islet Regeneration in the Post-Insulinoma NEDH Rat.

32. N. Sarvetnick, Islet cell destruction and regeneration in IFN-γ transgenic mice, J Cell Biochem. CB019:49 (abstract) (1991).

33. L. Rosenberg, W.P. Duguid, R.A. Brown, and A.I. Vinik, Induction of islet cell proliferation will reverse diabetes in the Syrian golden hamster, Diabetes. 37:334 (1988).

34. L. Rosenberg and A.I. Vinik, Regulation of pancreatic islet growth and differentiation: Evidence for paracrine and/or autocrine growth factor(s), Clin Res. 38:271A (1990).

35. L. Rosenberg and A.I. Vinik, In vitro stimulation of hamster pancreatic duct growth by an extract derived from the "wrapped" pancreas, (submitted for publication).

36. M.L. Brandi, G.D. Aurbach, L.A. Fitzpatrick, et al, Parathyroid mitogenic activity in plasma from patients with familial multiple endocrine neoplasia type 1, N Engl J Med. 314:1287-93 (1986).

37. S.J. Marx, K. Sakaguchi, J. Green, G.D. Aurbach, and M.L. Brandi, Mitogenic activity on parathyroid cells in plasma from members of a large kindred with multiple endocrine neoplasia Type 1, J Clin Endocrinol Metab. 67:149-53 (1988).

38. C. Larsson, B. Skogseid, K. Oberg, Y. Nakamura, and M. Nordenskjold, Multiple endocrine neoplasia type 1 gene maps to chromosome 11 and is lost in insulinoma, Nature. 332:85-87 (1988).

39. R.V. Thakker, P. Bouloux, C. Wooding, K. Chotai, P.M. Broad, N.K. Spurr, G.M. Besser, and J.L. O'Riordan, Association of parathyroid tumors in multiple endocrine neoplasia type 1 with loss of alleles on chromosome 11, N Engl J Med.321:218-24 (1989).

40. D. Owerbach, G.I. Bell, W.J. Rutter, J.A. Brown,and T.B. Shows, The insulin gene is activated on the short arm of chromosome 11 in humans, Diabetes. 30:267-70 (1981).

41. M.K. McLeod, A.M. Tutera, N.W. Thompson, and A.I. Vinik, Evidence for a pancreatic islet-cell mitogenic factor in patients with MEN-1, Association for Academic Surgery, Louisville, Kentucky, November 15-18, 1989.

SECTION ONE

REGULATION OF CELL GROWTH
AND DEVELOPMENT

THE ROLE OF GROWTH HORMONE AND PROLACTIN
IN BETA CELL GROWTH AND REGENERATION

Jens Høiriis Nielsen, Dr. Sc.,[1] Annette Møldrup, Ph.D.,[1]

Nils Billestrup, Ph.D.,[1] Elisabeth Douglas Petersen, M.Sc.,[1]

Giovanna Allevato, M.D.,[1] Matthias Stahl, M.D.[1]

[1]Hagedorn Research Laboratory

Gentofte, Denmark

INTRODUCTION

Although the natural history of Type I diabetes mellitus does not support a significant regenerative capacity of the pancreatic beta cell there is, however, evidence for a substantial postnatal enlargement of the beta cell mass in both rodent and man.[1,2] It was noted that the normal linear correlation between the logarithm of the body weight and the logarithm of the organ weight does not hold for the endocrine pancreas.[3] As shown schematically in Figure 1, the increase in the beta cell mass in the young rats lags behind that of the body weight, but catches up later in life. This may mean that the metabolic pressure on the beta cells during the rapid growth phase is not fully compensated for by a corresponding increase in the number of beta cells, which may explain the particular vulnerability of this cell type in childhood. During pregnancy there is a marked increase in the beta cell mass, which may reflect the increased demand for insulin during the considerable weight gain in the last trimester. In non-diabetic, obese humans, the islet mass is significantly greater than the islet mass of lean persons and that of obese patients with Type II diabetes.[4] Thus the striking coincidence of diabetes of either type with periods of accelerated growth of the body as summarized in Table 1, may lead to speculations of a connection between the beta cell number and the susceptibility to develop

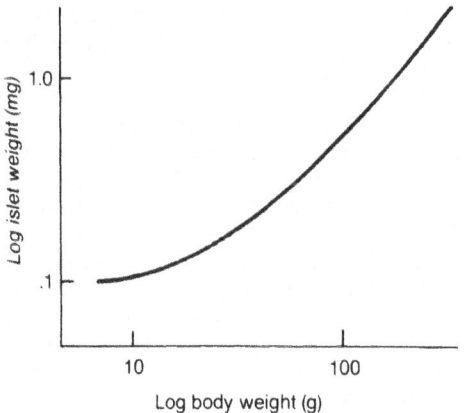

Figure 1. Schematic correlation between islet weight and body weight in a double logarithmic scale (adapted from reference 3).

Pancreatic Islet Cell Regeneration and Growth, Edited by A.I. Vinik
Plenum Press, New York, 1992

Table 1. Occurrence of Diabetes Mellitus under various conditions of growth.

Condition	DM Type	Hormonal Changes
Childhood	1	GH, IGF-I, T3
Puberty	1	GH, IGF-I, Sex Hormones
Pregnancy	GDM	PL, PRL, GH, Estrogens, Progesterone
Obesity	2	Adipsin, Incretin, IAPP(?)
Acromegaly	2	GH, IGF-I
Cushing's syndrome	2	Glucocorticods
Malnutrition	MRDM	Low IGF-I

GDM: gestational diabetes, MRDM: malnutrition related diabetes, GH: growth hormone, IGF: insulin-like growth factor, PL: placental lactogen, PRL: prolactin, IAPP: Islet-associated pancreatic protein

diabetes. Because the growth hormone family, including prolactin and placental lactogen, are involved in many growth processes this review focuses on the possible role of these hormones in the growth and regeneration of the endocrine pancreas.[5,6]

THE BETA CELL MASS AND DIABETES

Although chemically or surgically induced diabetes suggests that only 10 % of the beta cell mass is necessary for the maintenance of normal glucose tolerance other observations indicate that the total beta cell mass plays a role in the long-term regulation of the glucose metabolism. Thus 90% pancreatectomy or partial destruction of the beta cell by streptozotocin in neonatal rats results in later development of a Type II diabetes-like syndrome, in spite of considerable formation of new islets.[7] It is, however, in accordance with the recent report that removal of only half of the pancreas in man can cause impaired glucose tolerance.[8] In several genetically obese animals a marked hyperplasia of the beta cells is found. In spite of hyperinsulinemia glucose intolerance may develop, indicating either a primary functional defect of the secretory apparatus or a secondary effect due to insufficient growth of the beta cell mass in response to the vast increase in body mass. Support for the latter explanation is that restriction of the food intake will prevent the development of diabetes in the db/db mouse.[9] Also in type II diabetic patients with obesity weight reduction may lead to normalization of glucose metabolism.[2] Although it has not been proven that a reduced beta cell mass increases the susceptibility to develop type I diabetes, there is indirect evidence which supports this idea. Thus, reduced growth of the endocrine pancreas has been found in the prediabetic BB-rat.[10] Prophylactic treatment of such rats with insulin has been shown to postpone or prevent the development of diabetes,[11] which may be explained by protection of the reduced beta cell number against an autoimmune destruction. This is in accordance with the *in vitro* observation that stimulated beta cells are more susceptible to the toxic effect of interleukin-1 which has been implicated in the early destruction of beta cells leading to type I diabetes.[12] Lymphocytic infiltration of the islets may be genetically transmitted in these animal models, but this is not sufficient for beta cell destruction, as e.g., the male NOD mice have a low incidence of diabetes in spite of extensive lymphocytic infiltration of their islets.[13] Whether this depends on a sex-dependent difference in the beta cell number is not clear, but crosses between diabetes-prone BB rats and Zucker rats with hyperplastic islets are reported to have lymphocytic infiltration in the periphery of the giant islets, but do not develop Type I diabetes[14] indicating that the size of the beta cell mass may play a preventative role in the

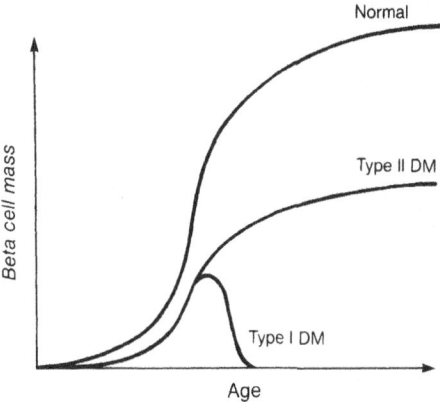

Figure 2. Hypothetical changes in the beta cell mass with age in normal and diabetic individuals, showing susceptibility of a reduced cell mass to autoimmune destruction in IDDM.

development of type I diabetes. It is thus hypothesized that a reduced number of beta cells increases the susceptibility to develop diabetes of either type as illustrated schematically in Figure 2.

GROWTH HORMONE, PROLACTIN AND PLACENTAL LACTOGEN, AND THE ENDOCRINE PANCREAS

Historically growth hormone (GH) is known for its diabetogenic effect by counteracting the effect of insulin on glucose metabolism. Thus, hypophysectomy leads to a marked increase in insulin sensitivity whereas growth hormone treatment results in insulin resistance and decreased glucose tolerance.[15] However, it was soon recognized that this diabetogenic effect was both age and species dependent. GH was found to be diabetogenic in adult dogs, but not in puppies and pregnant dogs,[16] and not in rats,[17] which may be explained by the ability of these animals to compensate for the increased insulin requirement by increasing the number of beta cells. Hyperglycemia has been described in acromegalic patients and individuals treated with GH,[18] whereas this has not been reported as a problem in GH-deficient children treated with GH.[19] Prolactin (PRL) and placental lactogen (PL) are also reported to exert insulin antagonistic effects and are supposed to play a role in the increased insulin demand during pregnancy.[20] Normally this is associated with a marked hyperplasia of the islets as demonstrated both in rats[21] and in women.[22] For a long time, however, this increase in the beta cell number was considered as secondary to the increased blood sugar level induced by these hormones, and only when techniques for maintaining isolated islets in culture became available[23] could direct trophic actions of the hormones be demonstrated, as is summarized in Table 2.

EFFECTS OF GH, PRL AND PL ON BETA CELLS IN VITRO

In addition to reports on the stimulation of insulin biosynthesis and secretion by GH in isolated islets we found that hGH, oPRL and hPL stimulated both insulin production and DNA synthesis in isolated islets from rats and mice maintained free-floating in culture in RPMI 1640 supplemented with a minimal amount of serum, i.e., 0.5%.[24] Although the effect of the hormones on the incorporation of tritiated thymidine (^{3}HTdR) into DNA was measurable after 6 to 12 hours the increases in insulin and DNA required days in culture.[25] Labelling of beta cell nuclei was found in monolayer cultures of neonatal rat pancreas exposed to GH.[26] In mouse islets a gradual reduction in the rate of insulin release was seen in the low serum containing medium and the hormone supplement prevented this decrease, whereas in rat islets the rate of release was constant at low serum and increased by the hormones.[5] In isolated islets from adult humans little or no stimulation was seen with hGH, although increased insulin

Table 2. Effects of Growth Hormone (GH), Prolactin (PRL) and Placental Lactogen (PL) on Pancreatic Islet Cells

Hormones	Observations	References
GH	Stimulation of insulin biosynthesis and secretion in rat islets	5
GH/PRL/PL	Stimulation of insulin secretion and DNA synthesis in cultured rat and mouse islets	24
GH	Stimulation of mitosis in beta cells in cultured rat pancreas	26
GH/PRL/PL	Stimulation of mitosis in beta cell in rat islet cell cultures	30
PRL	Stimulation of coupling between beta cells	29
GH	Stimulation of IGF-I production in fetal islets	52
GH	Stimulation of insulin mRNA in fetal human islets	57
PRL	Receptors in rat islets	32, 33
GH	Receptors in rat insulinoma cells	34
GH/PRL	Receptors in rat insulinoma cells similar to the cloned liver receptors	35

release was found in two cases where islets from children were exposed to hGH (unpublished observation). It should be mentioned that human islets have been reported to respond to the mitogenic effect of prolactin.[27] Since we found that hGH promoted the attachment and growth of dispersed newborn rat islet cells in monolayer culture we have employed a double immunocytochemical staining technique to identify the proliferating islet cells. We used monoclonal antibodies to bromodeoxyuridine (BrdU) to detect nuclei in S-phase and hormone antibodies to identify the cell type. We found that predominately insulin-containing cells incorporated BrdU in response to hGH, although both glucagon and somatostatin-containing cells remained in the cultures.[28] Pulse-chase experiments showed doublets of BrdU positive beta cells indicating that the cells had undergone mitosis. The increase in the number of beta cells was accompanied by a marked increase in the rate of insulin accumulation into the culture medium. During one to three months in culture a ten-fold increase in the insulin production could be observed. Although there was an increase in insulin biosynthesis by existing cells most of the long term increase in insulin production was due to an increase in cell number. These results suggest that GH acts both as a differentiation factor and as a growth factor for the beta cell. The effect on the glucose-stimulated insulin-release may be related to the increased coupling between the beta cells found in PRL treated islets.[29]

As hGH is known to react with both GH and PRL receptors in rodents we studied the effect of homologous hormones on beta cell proliferation. We found the same maximal effect of hGH, rGH, rPRL and hPL, but more rGH was required to obtain this effect.[30] This finding is in agreement with the higher potency of the lactogenic hormones on rat islets reported recently,[31] but it may, however, also reflect a lower potency or stability of the rat GH preparation.

EXPRESSION OF GH AND PRL RECEPTORS ON INSULIN PRODUCING CELLS

Normal adult rat islets seem predominantly to express lactogenic receptors[32] as seen by in situ hormone binding to pancreas sections[33] and by immunocytochemical staining with antibodies to PRL and GH receptors. (Unpublished observation) However the differential expression of the two receptor types may vary with age and physiological state of the animal as well as the *in vitro* conditions. By binding studies,[34] affinity cross-linking and mRNA analysis we have identified GH and PRL receptors similar to those cloned from the liver in the rat insulinoma cell line RIN 5AH.[35] Transfection of these cells with the cloned rat GH receptor cDNA confers increased responsiveness to the insulinotrophic action of GH indicating that the cloned receptor is functioning in insulin producing cells.[36] Several forms of both GH and PRL receptors have been described,[37] although only one gene for each has been found. The long and the short forms of the receptors may have different functions. Thus, we found that a truncated form of the growth hormone receptor lacking about half of the cytoplasmatic domain was unable to transmit the insulinotrophic signal, but was still able to bind and internalize GH.[38] Similarly only the long form of the PRL receptor was found to induce transcription of beta lactoglobulin.[39] We are presently studying the regulation of the expression of the long and short forms of the GH and PRL receptors in normal islets.

ROLE OF PL, PRL AND GH IN ISLET GROWTH DURING PREGNANCY

The dramatic rise in PL during the last trimester and the rise in PRL during pregnancy and lactation, in combination with the above mentioned stimulatory effects on beta cell growth and function, suggests that these hormones may be involved in the beta cell hyperplasia in pregnancy. In rodents there are two placental lactogens that may play distinct roles.[40] A role of GH can, however, not be excluded since a variant GH gene is being expressed in the human placenta, and the hormone vGH is apparently the dominant form of circulating GH during pregnancy.[41] We have cultured mouse islets in medium supplemented with 10% serum from women in the last trimester and found a significant increase in the DNA content, but a decrease in the insulin content. Having previously shown that exposure of islets to progesterone results in an *increased* sensitivity to glucose, but a *decrease* in the stored insulin, we cultured the islets with either PL or progesterone and a combination of both. In concentrations similar to those found in pregnant serum, PL counteracted the progesterone-induced decrease in insulin content,[42] suggesting that PL may be responsible for the beta cell hyperplasia in pregnancy. In addition, the responsiveness of the beta cell to the trophic hormones may be determined by the level of expression of the receptors, which is currently being investigated. Thus pregnancy offers a unique opportunity to study beta cell growth and regeneration because it represents a state in which unresponsive adult beta cells become responsive to gestational growth promoting hormones.

ROLE OF GH AND PRL IN BETA CELL REGENERATION IN DIABETES

The diabetogenic properties of GH and PRL do not indicate any therapeutic role in the treatment of diabetes, unless beta cells exposed to destructive agents become sensitized to the trophic hormones. Alternatively, it may be that the toxic agents result in loss of sensitivity to the trophic hormones leading to rapid disappearance of the beta cells. In an attempt to elucidate these possibilities we have exposed newborn rat islets *in vitro* to agents known to be toxic to beta cells *in vivo* and *in vitro*, namely streptozotocin (STZ) and interleukin-1.(IL-1). After loss of about 80% of the beta cells, the remaining islets were cultured for two weeks in the presence of hGH. The insulin release to the medium and the insulin and DNA content of the islets were determined. Whereas the islets treated with IL-1 responded normally to hGH, the STZ treated islets showed an additional loss of beta cells when exposed to hGH.[43,44] It has recently been reported that the mitogenic response to amniotic fluid was also lost after STZ treatment.[45] These results indicate that the cytotoxic mechanisms differ between these two agents. In accordance with current theories, STZ induces DNA strand breaks, which *do not* abolish the ability to make insulin,[46] but *do* prevent the mitotic capacity of islet cells. On the other hand IL-1 may preferentially kill the terminally differentiated beta cells and may leave the less differentiated, but mitotically active precursor cells intact, or even stimulate their growth.[47,48] If these preliminary *in vitro* results can be extrapolated into the *in vivo* situation, it may be speculated that with certain types of diabetes the capacity to regeneration via proliferation of surviving beta cells is lost, whereas in other forms the remaining cells may proliferate in response to appropriate growth factors. In Type I diabetes, however, the immune system may destroy regenerated beta cells. Therefore, either suppression of the autoimmune reaction or enhancement of beta cell regeneration may have therapeutic relevance. The remarkable islet neogenesis found in the transgenic mouse model of autoimmune diabetes[49] indicates a regenerative potential in adult animals, which is also supported by other models such as the rats with insulinoma-suppressed islets[50] or duct-ligated pancreas.[51] The role that growth hormone plays in beta cell regeneration is, as yet, speculative. It may be that the pancreas will react to injury by regenerative processes like the liver, where partial hepatectomy is followed by a marked hypertrophy of the somatotrophs,[52] implicating involvement of GH in the regenerative process. It is noteworthy that islet cell hyperplasia has been described in cases of liver damage.[53]

INSULIN AS A SOMATOMEDIN

In the search for the mechanism of action of GH on the beta cell we have looked for a role of IGF-I as a mediator of the action of GH. By adding neutralizing antiserum to IGF-I we were not able to block the mitogenic effect of GH and addition of IGF-I did not affect mitotic activity. By Northern blot analysis of 20 μg polyA RNA of GH-stimulated islets we could not detect any IGF-I mRNA[30] in agreement with recent in situ hybridization data.[54] In addition, PRL and PL , which have the same effect on the beta cells as GH, are not supposed to act via IGF-I. Thus our results indicate that GH, PRL and PL act directly on the beta cell, independent of IGF-I. IGF-I may, however, play a role in the growth of the fetal pancreas.[55,56] Although receptors for IGF-I are present on adult beta cells they may not transmit a mitogenic signal but rather mediate an inhibitory effect on insulin secretion.[57,58] Although insulin is expressed in the absence of GH, GH has a marked stimulatory effect on the insulin mRNA level as demonstrated in RIN 5AH cells, rat islets[60] and fetal human islets.[61] We are currently looking for a GH responsive element in the 5'-flanking region of the insulin gene. GH seems not to stimulate the expression of the proto-oncogenes c-fos and c-jun in RIN cells[59,62] although it may do so in other cell types.[63] On the basis of the homology between insulin and the IGFs and the responsiveness of beta cells to GH, insulin may be considered as a somatomedin. This is further supported by the essential role of insulin in the growth-promoting effect of GH in vivo. Diabetic animals do not grow in response to GH unless insulin is administered concomitantly.[64] Thus insulin may be included in a key position of the regulatory pathway of growth control as depicted in Figure 3. To the upper right is indicated that PL may regulate IGF II production during fetal growth and together with PRL increase the insulin supply both in the fetus and the mother via the lactogenic receptors (PRL-R) and a putative PL-R. To the upper left is shown that GH stimulates postnatal growth through its receptor (GH-R) modulated by the circulating binding protein GH-BP as well as via IGF I and the indispensable role for insulin. The fact that the beta cells respond to both somatogenic and lactogenic hormones may explain why patients with Laron-type dwarfism lacking the growth hormone receptor[65] and/or IGF I production do not have diabetes. Similarly the Snell dwarf mouse which lacks both GH and PRL in the pituitary due to a mutation in the gene for the transcription factor Pit-1/GHF-1[66] is not born with diabetes probably due to normal expression of the placental hormones.

IS THE BETA CELL MASS DETERMINED PRENATALLY?

We are still faced with the question: What determines the beta cell mass? There are certain indications for a role of genetic factors in the replication capacity of the beta cells in various strains of mice.[67] However environmental factors like nutrition during fetal development may also play an important role. Thus morphological studies of the pancreas in the offspring of rats on a protein-depleted diet during pregnancy showed a marked reduction in the ratio between islet volume and body weight.[68] This may explain the development of certain forms of malnutrition-related diabetes mellitus (MRDM).[69] In this connection it may be of considerable interest that a correlation between birth weight and glucose tolerance years later has been found in a population study,[70] which may suggest that growth and development of the endocrine pancreas may be retarded by the lack of proper nutrients. Although serum GH often is elevated in malnutrition the IGF-1 level is low and it was recently reported that there is a reduction of GH receptor expression in certain tissues.[71] Recently GH receptor mRNA was detected in fetal human pancreas,[72] and we are currently investigating the expression of GH

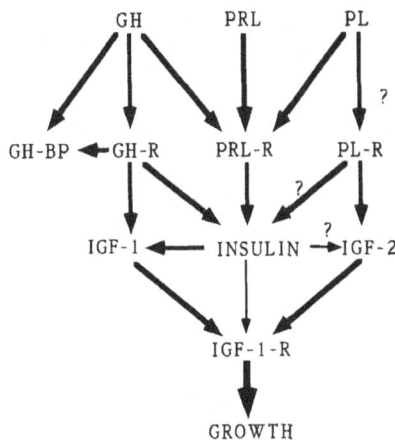

Figure 3. Hypothetical interactions between peptide hormones and receptors involved in somatic growth (see text).

and PRL receptors during the embryogenesis of the mouse pancreas. In the future it will be interesting to see if members of this family of hormones play a role in the differentiation of stem cells in the duct epithelium into insulin-producing islet cells, and whether it may become possible to induce formation of new beta cells later in life.

ACKNOWLEDGEMENTS

The authors want to thank the Juvenile Diabetes Foundation, the Danish Research Council for Health Sciences, the Danish Research Academy and the Swiss National Science Foundation and the school of Medicine, University of Catanzoro, Italy for financial support.

REFERENCES

1. J. Logothetopoulos, Islet cell regeneration and neogenesis, *in:* "Handbook of Physiology, Sect. 7, vol. 1.", D.F. Steiner and N. Freinkel, eds., American Physiological Society, Washington, D.C. pp 67-76 (1972).
2. C. Hellerström, I. Swenne, and A.Andersson, *in:* "The Pathology of the endocrine Pancreas in Diabetes," P.J. Lefebvre and D.G. Pipeleers, eds. Springer Verlag, Berlin, pp. 141-170 (1988).
3. B. Hellman, The total volume of the pancreatic islet tissue at different ages of the rat, APMIS. 47:35-50 (1959).
4. J. Rahier, The diabetic pancreas: A pathologist's view, in: "The Pathology of the endocrine pancreas in diabetes," P.J. Lefebvre and D.G. Pipeleers, eds., Springer Verlag, Berlin. pp. 17-40 (1988).
5. J.H. Nielsen, Growth and function of the pancreatic β cell *in vitro*. Effects of glucose hormones and serum factors on mouse, rat and human pancreatic islets in organ culture, Acta Endocrinol (Copenh). 108 (suppl 266):1-39 (1985).
6. J.J. Nielsen, Å. Lernmark, O.D. Madsen, B.S. Welinder, S. Linde, N. Billestrup, and A. Moldrup, Effects of growth hormone on the endocrine pancreas, *in:* "Growth hormone, basic and clinical aspects", O. Isaksson, B. Hokfeldt, and C. Binder, eds., Nordisk Insulin Symposium No. 1. Excerpta Medica Int. Congr. Ser. No. 748, Amsterdam, pp. 227-237 (1987).
7. G.C. Weir, J.L. Leahy, and S. Bonner-Weir, Experimental reduction of β-cell mass: Implications for the pathogenesis of diabetes, Diabetes Metab Rev. 2:125-161 (1986).
8. D.M. Kendall, D.E.R. Sutherland, J.S. Najarian, F.C. Goetz, and R.P. Robertson, Effects of hemipancreatectomy on insulin secretion and glucose tolerance in healthy humans, N Engl J Med. 322:898-903 (1990).
9. W.L. Chick and A.A. Like, Studies in the diabetic mutant mouse. III. Physiological factors associated with alterations in beta-cell proliferation, Diabetologia. 6:243-51 (1970).
10. M. Löhr M, H. Markholst, T. Dyrberg, G. Klöppel, M. Oberholzer, and Å. Lernmark, Insulitis and diabetes are preceded by a decrease in ß cell volume in diabetes-prone BB rats, Pancreas. 3:140-44 (1988).
11. C.F. Godtfredsen, K. Buschard, and E.K. Frandsen, Reduction of diabetes incidence of BB Wistar rats by early prophylactic insulin treatment of diabetes-prone animals, Diabetologia. 28:933-35 (1985).

12. T. Mandrup-Poulsen, S. Helqvist, L.D. Wogensen, J. Molvig, F. Pociot, J. Johannesen, and J. Nerup, Cytokines and free radicals as effector molecules in the destruction of pancreatic beta cells, *in:* "Human Diabetes. Curr Top Microbiol Immunol Vol 164," S. Baekkskov and B. Hansen, eds., Springer Verlag, Berlin pp. 169-193 (1990).

13. T. Hanafusa and S. Tarui, Immune pathogenesis of diabetes in the nonobese diabetic mouse: An overview," *in:* "The Role of Viruses and the Immune System in Diabetes Mellitus. Curr Top Microbiol Immunol Vol 156," Dryberg, ed., Springer Verlag, Berlin pp. 15-25 (1990).

14. D.L. Guberski, L. Butler, and A.A. Like, The BBZ/Wor rat: pancreatic β-cells of obese rats are more susceptible to immune destruction than B cells of lean rats, *in:* "Frontiers in diabetes research: Lessons from animal diabetes, volume 2," E. Shafrir and A.E. Renold, eds., J Libbey, New York pp. 268-272 (1988).

15. M.B. Davidson, Effect of growth hormone on carbohydrate and lipid metabolism, Endocr Rev. 8:115-31 (1987).

16. F.G. Young and A. Korner, Growth hormone, *in:* "Diabetes", R.H. Williams, ed., Paul B Hoeber, New York pp. 216-237 (1960).

17. B.A. Houssay, Other hormones, *in:* "Diabetes", R.H. Williams, ed., Paul B Hoeber, New York pp. 233-256 (1960).

18. E. Cerasi and R. Luft, Human growth hormone as a regulator of blood glucose concentrations and as a diabetogenic substance, Lancet. 2:1359-61 (1963).

19. J. Walker, J.L. Chaussain, and P.F. Bougneres, Growth hormone treatment of children with short stature increases insulin secretion but does not impair glucose disposal, J Clin Endocrinol Metab. 69: 253-58 (1989).

20. N. Freinkel, Of pregnancy and progeny, Diabetes. 29:1023-35 (1980).

21. I.C. Green, S. ElSeifi, D. Perrin, and S.L. Howell, Cell replication in the islets of Langerhans of adult rats: effects of pregnancy, ovariectomy and treatment with steroid hormones, J Endocrinol. 54:317-25 (1981).

22. F.A. VanAssche, L. Aerts, and F. DePrins, A morphological study of the endocrine pancreas in human pregnancy, Br J Obstet Gynaecol. 85:818-20 (1978).

23. A. Andersson and C. Hellerstöm, Metabolic characteristics of isolated pancreatic islets in tissue culture, Diabetes. 21(suppl 2):546-54 (1972).

24. J.H. Nielsen, Effects of growth hormone, prolactin and placental lactogen on insulin content and release and deoxyribonucleic acid synthesis in cultured pancreatic islets, Endocrinology. 110:600-06 (1982).

25. J.H. Nielsen, Hormonal regulation of growth and function of insulin producing cells in culture, *in:* "Hormonally defined media: A tool in cell biology," G. Fischer and R.J. Wieser, eds., Springer Verlag, Berlin pp. 264-274 (1983).

26. A. Rabinovitch, C. Quigley, and M.W. Rechler MW, Growth hormone stimulates islet β-cell replication in neonatal rat pancreatic monolayer culture, Diabetes. 32:307-12 (1983).

27. R.L. Sorenson, "Islet β-cell division during pregnancy. a role for lactogenic hormones," Lecture at: Pancreatic Beta-Cell 1991: Gene to Disease. Joslin Diabetes Center, Boston. June 29-July 1, 1991

28. J.H. Nielsen, S. Linde, B.S. Welinder, N. Billestrup, and O.D. Madsen, Growth hormone is a growth factor for the differentiated pancreatic β-cell, Mol Endocrinol. 3:165-73 (1989).

29. R.L. Sorenson, T.C. Brelje, O.D. Hegre, S. Marshall, P. Anaya, and J.D. Sheridan, Prolactin (*in vitro*) decreases the glucose stimulation, enhances insulin secretion, and increases dye coupling among islet B cells, Endocrinology. 121:1447-53 (1987).

30. N. Billestrup and J.H. Nielsen, The stimulatory effect of growth hormone, prolactin and placental lactogen on β-cell proliferation is not mediated by insulin-like growth factor-I, Endocrinology. 129:883-88 (1991).

31. T.C. Brelje, P. Allaire, O. Hegre, and R.L. Sorenson, Effect of prolactin versus growth hormone on islet function and the importance of using homologous mammosomatotropic hormones, Endocrinology. 125:2392-99 (1989).

32. M. Tessone, R. Oliveira-Filho, and E.H. Charreau, Prolactin binding in rat Langerhans islets, J Recept Res. 1:355-82 (1980).

33. M. Polak, R. Scharfmann, E. Ban, F. Haour, M.C. Postel-Vinay, and P. Czernichow, Demonstration of lactogenic receptors in rat endocrine pancreases by quantitative autoradiography, Diabetes. 39:1045-49 (1990).

34. N. Billestrup and J.M. Martin, Growth hormone binding to specific receptors stimulates growth and function of cloned insulin-producing rat insulinoma RIN-5AH cells, Endocrinology. 116:1175-81 (1985).

35. A. Möldrup, N. Billestrup, and J.H. Nielsen, Rat insulinoma cells express both a 115 kDa GH receptor and a 95 kDa PRL-receptor structurally related to the cloned hepatic receptors, J Biol Chem. 265:8686-90 (1990).

36. N. Billestrup, A. Möldrup, P. Serup, L.S. Mathews, G. Norstedt, and J.H. Nielsen, Introduction of exogenous growth hormone receptors augments growth hormone responsive insulin biosynthesis in rat insulinoma cells, Proc Natl Acad Sci USA. 87:7210-14 (1990).

37. A. Möldrup, N. Billestrup, A. Thorn, Å. Lernmark, and J.H. Nielsen, Multiple growth hormone-binding proteins are expressed on insulin-producing cells, Mol Endocrinol. 3:1173-82 (1989).

38. A. Moldrup, G. Allevato, T. Dyrberg, J.H. Nielsen, and N. Billestrup, Growth hormone action in rat insulinoma cells expressing truncated growth hormone receptors, J Biol Chem. 266:17440-45 (1991).

39. L. Lesueur, M. Edery, S. Ali, J. Paly, P.A. Kelly, J. Djiane, Comparison of long and short forms of the prolactin receptor on prolactin-induced milk protein gene transcription, Proc Natl Acad Sci USA. 88:824-28 (1991).

40. T.C. Brelje and R.L. Sorenson, Role of prolactin versus growth hormone on islet B-cell proliferation *in vitro*: Implications for pregnancy, Endocrinology. 128:45-57 (1991).

41. J.N. MacLeod, I. Worsley, J. Ray, H.G. Friesen, S.A. Liebhaber, and N.E. Cooke, Human growth hormone-variant is a biologically active somatogen and lactogen, Endocrinology. 128:1298-1302 (1991).

42. J.H. Nielsen, V. Nielsen, L.M. Pedersen, and T. Deckert, Effects of pregnancy hormones on pancreatic islets in organ culture, Acta Endocrinol (Copenh). 111:336-41 (1986).
43. J.H. Nielsen, D. Jensen, and R. Jorgensen, Impairment of the β-cell response to growth hormone after streptozotocin treatment of rat islets *in vitro*, Diabetologia. 32:522A (1989).
44. M. Stahl and J.H. Nielsen, Effects of IL-1 and hGH on the DNA synthesis of rat pancreatic beta cells in culture, Diabetologia.34 (suppl 2):A95 (1991).
45. A. Dunger, A. Sjöholm, and D.L. Eizirik, Amino acids and human amniotic fluid increase DNA biosynthesis in pancreatic islets of adult mouse, but this effect is lost following exposure to streptozotocin, Pancreas. 5:639-46 (1990).
46. N. Welsh and C. Hellerstrom, Invitro restoration of insulin production in islets from adult rats treated neonatally with streptozotocin, Endocrinology. 126:1842-1848 (1990).
47. M. Stahl, R.O. Petersen, and J.H. Nielsen, Effect of interleukin-1 on 5-bromodeoxydine incorporation into rat pancreatic beta cells in culture, Diabetes. 40(suppl 1):151A (1991).
48. A. Sjoholm, Long-term regulation of pancreatic β-cell replication and insulin secretion by cytokines and adrenergic agents, Diabetologia. 34(suppl 2):A94 (1991).
49. N.E. Sarvetnick, This Volume.
50. C. Newgard, This Volume.
51. L. Rosenberg, This Volume.
52. J.M.E. Llanos, C.L.G. Dumm, and A.C. Nessi,, Ultrastucture of STH cells of the pars distalis of hepatectomized mice, Z Zellforsch. 113:29-38 (1971).
53. W. Gepts and P.M. LeCompte, "The pathology of type I (juvenile) diabetes," *in:* " The diabetic pancreas. Second edition", B.W. Volk and ER. Arquilla, eds., Plenum, New York (1985).
54. F.E. Smith, K.M. Rosen, L. Villa-Komarov, G.C. Weir, and S. Bonner-Weir, Enhanced insulin-like growth factor I gene expression in regenerating rat pancreas. Proc Natl Acad Sci USA 88:6152-6156 (1991).
55. I. Swenne, D.J. Hill, A.J. Strain, and R.D.G. Milner, Effects of human placental lactogen and growth hormone on the production of insulin and somatomedin C/insulin-like growth factor I by human fetal pancreas in tissue culture, J Endocrinol. 113:297-303 (1987).
56. D.J. Hill, This Volume.
57. C.F.H. Van Schravendijk, L. Heylen, J.L. Van den Brande, and D.G. Pipeleers, Direct effect of insulin and insulin-like growth factor-I on the secretory activity of rat pancreatic beta cells, Diabetologia. 33:649-53 (1990).
58. J.L. Leahy and K.M. Van DeKerkhove, Insulin-like growth factor I at physiological concentrations is a potent inhibitor of insulin secretion, Endocrinology. 126:1593-98 (1990).
59. E.D. Pedersen, N. Billestrup, and J.H. Nielsen, Effect of growth hormone and serum on the expression of the proto-oncogenes c-jun and c-fos in insulin produing cells, Biomed Biochim Acta. 49(12):1269-73 (1990).
60. J. Brunstedt, Expression of the insulin gene: Regulation by glucose, hydrocortisone and growth hormone in mouse pancreatic islets in organ culture, Acta Biol Med Germ. 41:1151-55 (1982).
61. B. Formby, A. Ullrich, L. Coussens, L. Walker, and C.M. Peterson, Growth hormone stimulates insulin gene expression in cultured human fetal pancreatic islets, J Clin Endocrinol Metab. 66:1075-79 (1988).
62. M. Asfari, B. Breant, and G. Rosselin, Induction of DNA synthesis and gene expression by human growth hormone in a highly differentiated rat insulinoma cell culture, Diabetes. 40(suppl 1):215A (1991).
63. M.C. Slootweg, R.P. deGroot, M.P.M. Herrmann-Erlee, I. Koornneef, W. Kruijer, and Y.M. Kramer, Growth hormone induces expression of c-jun and jun B oncogenes and employs a protein kinase C signal transduction pathway for the induction of c-fos oncogene expression, J Mol Endocrinol. 6:179-88 (1991).
64. R.O. Scow, Effect of growth hormone on growth in hypophysectomized-pancreactomized rats, Endocrinology. 61:582-86 (1957).
65. P.J. Godowski, D.W. Leung, L.R. Meacham, J.P. Galgani, R. Hellmiss, R. Keret, P.S. Rotwein, J.S. Parks, Z. Laron, and W.I. Wood, Characterization of the human growth hormone receptor gene and demonstration of a partial gene deletion in two patients with Laron-type dwarfism, Proc Natl Acad Sci USA. 86:8083-87 (1989).
66. S. Li, E.B. Crenshaw, E.J. Rawson, D.M. Simmons, L.W. Swanson, and M.G. Rosenfeld, Dwarf locus mutants lacking three pituitary cell types results from mutations in the POU-domain gene pit-1, Nature. 347:528-33 (1990).
67. I. Swenne and A. Andersson, Effect of genetic background on the capacity for islet cell replication in mice, Diabetologia. 27:464-67 (1984).
68. C. Weinkowe, E. Weinkowe, A. Timme, and B. Pimstone, Pancreatic islets of malnourished rats: quantitative histologic and electron microscopy findings, Arch Pathol Lab Med. 101:266-69 (1977).
69. P.J. Lefebvre, Clinical forms of diabetes mellitus, *in:* "The pathology of the endocrine pancreas," P.J. Lefebvre and D.G. Pipeleers, eds., Springer Verlag, Berlin pp. 1-16 (1988).
70. C.N. Hales, Non-insulin dependent diabetes mellitus - the thrifty phenotype? Lecture at: 27th Annual Meeting of the European Association for the Study of Diabetes. Dublin, Ireland. Sept. 10-14, 1991.
71. M. Maes, D. Maiter, J.P. Thissen, L.E. Underwood, and J.M. Ketelslegers, Contributions of growth hormone receptor and postreceptor defects to growth hormone resistance in malnutrition, Trends Endocrinol Metab. 2:92-97 (1991).
72. P.J. Miettinen, T. Otonkoski, and R. Voutilainen, "Regulation of insulin and IGF-II mRNA expression in human fetal pancreas islets", 2nd International Symposium on Insulin-like Growth Factors/Somatomedins. San Francisco. Jan 12-16, 1991. Abstracts (p. 160).

DISCUSSION

D. LeRoith: In your studies on the islet cells have you excluded a paracrine effect on the endocrine cells? Could the growth hormone be acting on them to send a signal to the islet cells?

J. Nielsen: Yes, we have excluded a paracrine effect of growth hormone. Actually, in our cultures we have almost all endocrine cells. Sometimes there are a few fibroblasts, but in most cases they are only endocrine cells. We can account for all the cells by staining with insulin, glucagon, and somatostatin. There is no growth hormone.

D. LeRoith: So it is still possible that, *in vivo*, growth hormone could be working as an endocrine factor through other cells to stimulate pancreatic growth. In other words, there could be multiple factors activated by growth hormone.

J. Nielsen: On the other hand, from the staining with receptor antibodies, it looks as though the highest density of cells are endocrine islet cells, but we cannot exclude the possibility that there are other cells which growth hormone targets.

S. Bonner-Weir: You made the comment about the absence of blood cells ... But there is blood going to the islet and then from the islet to the the exocrine tissue. Would this counteract the likelihood that you would have paracrine flow from the exocrine tissue to the islet cells?

J. Nielsen: The direction of bloodflow suggests that there maybe a substance coming from the endocrine to the exocrine cells. Paracrine flow would be through the interstitium between the cells, but it could still flow back.

S. Bonner-Weir: You could have some flow from the islet to acinar cells, but not the corollary. There is a very thin capsule around the islets, of fibroblasts and collagen on the outside, within the capsule. This may act as a barrier to the flow from acinar cells to the islet.

C. Newgard: Jens, I was just curious about how you control for insulin accumulation while you are doing growth hormone incubation. I presume that a cell incubated in growth hormone would tend to accumulate insulin faster. A second, point relates to is what glucose concentration you are using because you could potentially separate the effects you're seeing into a glucose sensing effect versus an islet number effect?

J. Nielsen: We have the stimulatory effect - the concentration is 11 millimolar glucose in the medium, but we have looked at the acute effects of glucose and the islets exposed to growth hormone and it doesn't look like they become more sensitive to glucose. We get a higher maximal effect, but the sensitivity is not increased.

C. Newgard: It's remarkable that if insulin is, indeed, higher in growth hormone treated experiments, insulin would tend to down regulate insulin content, yet you are still seeing the effect. If you control for insulin would you see any greater effect?

J. Nielsen: I don't think so. I mean, I don't believe in the "defective" effect of insulin because some years ago, we studied the effects of very huge doses of insulins on the C-peptide secretion from human islets and we didn't see any effects.

THE INSULIN-LIKE GROWTH FACTOR FAMILY OF
PEPTIDES, BINDING PROTEINS AND RECEPTORS:
THEIR POTENTIAL ROLE IN TISSUE REGENERATION

Derek LeRoith, M.D., Ph.D.,[1] Haim Werner, Ph.D.,[1]

Bartolome Burguera M.D., Ph.D.,[1] Charles T. Roberts, Jr., Ph.D.,[1]

Susan Mulroney, Ph.D.,[2] and Aviad Haramati, Ph.D.[2]

[1] NIH - Diabetes Branch

Section on Molecular and Cellular Physiology

Bethesda, MD 20892

[2] Georgetown University

Department of Physiology

Washington, DC 20007

INTRODUCTION

The insulin-like growth factors (IGF-I and IGF-II) are mitogenic peptides that are structurally related to insulin (Figure 1). Until recently, these growth factors were thought to be produced exclusively by the liver and to act solely in an endocrine manner.[1-3] According to the "somatomedin hypothesis," the synthesis of IGF-I by the liver and its secretion are regulated by growth hormone (GH) and, following its release into the circulation, IGF-I reaches its target tissues where it induces growth and development, thereby mediating the effect of GH during the growth period.

Over the past decade, numerous studies have demonstrated that, while the liver produces the majority of circulating IGF-I and IGF-II, most, if not all, extrahepatic tissues also synthesize these growth factors at various developmental stages.

Interestingly, the extrahepatic production of the IGFs, though somewhat affected by GH, is generally more highly regulated by other tissue specific factors. For example, IGF-I gene expression in the ovary is regulated by estrogens and in bone by parathyroid hormone and estrogen. Presumably the IGFs produced in extrahepatic tissues remain in the local environment and therefore function locally via paracrine or autocrine mechanisms. The effects of locally produced IGFs, in addition to growth of tissues, also include cellular differentiation.[1-3]

The biological effects of the IGFs are mediated by specific cell surface receptors. These include the IGF-I receptor, the insulin receptor, and the IGF-II/mannose-6-phosphate (m-6-p) receptor. The IGF-I and insulin receptors are structurally very similar, although they are the products of separate genes located on different chromosomes. They both consist of two alpha subunits and two beta subunits joined by disulfide linkages to form a heterotetrameric complex (Figure 2). The alpha subunits lie entirely extracellularly and bind the ligands, whereas the beta subunits anchor the receptor in the membrane and their cytoplasmic domains display tyrosine kinase activity. In contrast, the IGF-II/M-6-P receptor has a totally

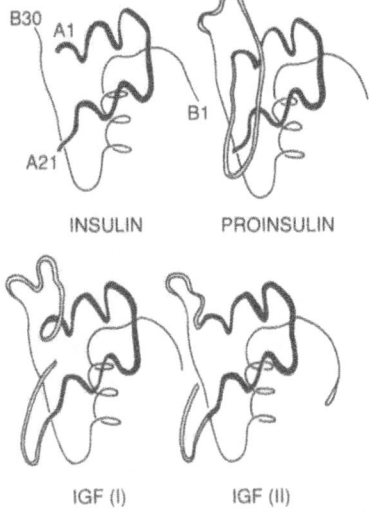

INSULIN   PROINSULIN

IGF (I)   IGF (II)

Figure 1. Tertiary structure of the insulin-like growth factor family of peptides.

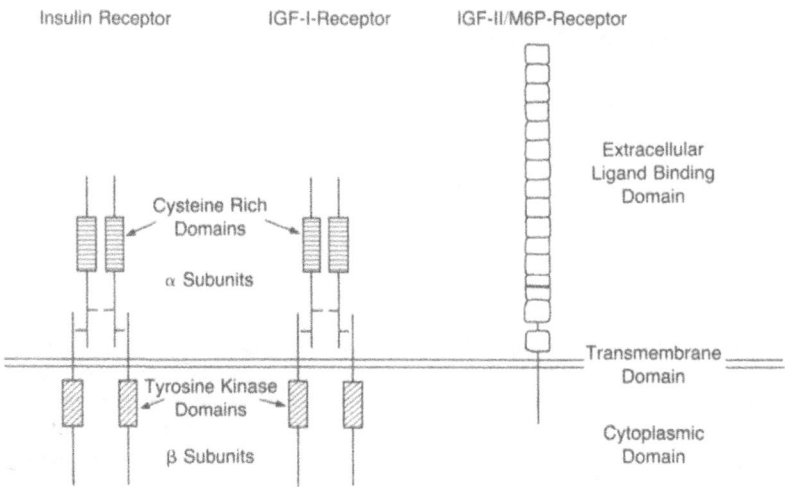

Figure 2. Schematic representation of the insulin-like growth factor family of receptors.

different structure, consisting of multiple extracellular repeats with a very short cytoplasmic domain which lacks kinase activity. The IGF-I receptor exhibits high affinity binding to IGF-I and IGF-II, as does the IGF-II/M-6-P receptor. Insulin can bind to the IGF-I receptor with a lower affinity, but does not bind to the IGF-II/M-6-P receptor. Whereas the IGF-I receptor mediates many of the biological functions of the IGFs, presumably via tyrosine kinase activity, the IGF-II/M-6-P receptor was for a long time thought to be incapable of mediating these effects. Recently, however, studies by Nishimoto and colleagues have suggested that the IGF-II/M-6-P (M-6-P) receptor may play a role in signal transduction in certain cells, possibly by affecting Ca^{++} fluxes through coupling to G proteins.[4]

The IGFs circulate complexed with specific IGF binding proteins (IGF-BPs). These binding proteins, of which 6 have been identified and characterized, have a number of important functions. In the circulation, IGF-BPs prolong the half-life of IGF's, prevent IGF from interacting with insulin receptors and deliver circulating IGFs to their target tissues. At the local tissue level, IGF-BPs apparently regulate the biological functions of the IGFs. In general, they have been shown to inhibit the biological actions of the IGFs. However, under certain conditions they enhance their effects.[5]

The functions of this complex family of growth factors, binding proteins and receptors in individual tissues are highly specific. For example, in the nervous system, IGFs act as neurotrophic factors, in the reproductive system they enhance steroidogenesis, and in the skeletal system they are important in maintaining normal bone density. In this review, we will explore the possible roles of the IGFs and their receptors in tissue growth and regeneration.

COMPENSATORY RENAL GROWTH (CRG) FOLLOWING UNILATERAL NEPHRECTOMY (UNX) AS A MODEL FOR CELL GROWTH

The Role of GH in Renal Growth

It is well-known that removal of one kidney results, within days, in accelerated growth of the contralateral (remaining) kidney. In adult animals, the increase in renal mass is primarily due to hypertrophy, i.e., an increase in cell size and tubule length, whereas in immature animals, growth occurs largely by hyperplasia, i.e., cell multiplication.[6] Some of the initial events in the cellular response to UNX include increases in single nephron glomerular filtration rate and tubular ion transport systems and sensitization of the renal tubule to renal growth factors. A fundamental question, as yet unanswered, is whether the mechanisms governing the CRG are entirely locally mediated or whether they also involve other circulating hormonal factors such as GH. Hypophysectomy slows CRG after UNX, suggesting that GH may play a role in this model of renal growth.[7] The possible relevance of changes in circulating pulsatile GH in the initial CRG following unilateral nephrectomy was recently assessed in adult male Wistar rats.[8] The animals were implanted with silastic jugular catheters and underwent either UNX (with adrenal glands remaining intact) or a sham operation (where the kidney was manipulated but not removed). Following surgery, blood samples were obtained every 15 min over a 6-hr period from conscious unrestrained rats. The adult UNX rats demonstrated a significant increase in GH levels within 24 hrs after surgery. Peak GH levels were 4-fold greater in UNX rats (417 ± 75 ng/ml) as compared with control rats (119 ± 23 ng/ml) ($p < 0.05$). The rise in GH release appeared to be transient since by 48 hrs this increase waned. To examine whether the increase in GH release is involved in the initial CRG, an antagonist to GH-releasing factor, (GRF-AN:(N-Ac- Tyr-Arg)-GRF-(1-29)-NH_2, which successfully blocks GH release in immature and adult rats, was used to block the increase in GH levels 24 hours post-UNX. Rats underwent UNX following which they were injected with the GRF-AN (200 ug/kg twice daily) and GH levels were analyzed during 24 hrs post-surgery.[9] GH levels were almost totally suppressed and CRG was markedly attenuated, supporting the hypothesis that GH is indeed involved in the initial growth response of the remnant kidney in adult rats.[10]

In contrast, studies in immature rats suggested that the initial CRG seen within 24 hrs of UNX is not GH-dependent. Injection of GRF-AN in immature rats caused an attenuation of body growth, but had minimal effect on growth of the remnant kidney. Thus, the mechanisms involved in causing CRG in immature rats may differ from those causing hypertrophy in adult rats and GH appears to be implicated only in the latter.

The Role Of Insulin-like Growth Factors

Since IGF-I mediates many, if not most, of the growth-promoting actions of GH *and* IGF-II is also mitogenic, although less GH-dependent, the role of these growth factors in CRG was studied. Administration of IGF-I to rats and man increases glomerular filtration rate and renal plasma flow, and injection of IGF-I into hypophysectomized rats causes kidney growth.[11,12] Although there is a consensus that renal tissue IGF-I levels increase 3-5 days following UNX in adult rats, the question remains as to whether this increase is associated with a prior increase in kidney IGF-I gene expression or whether this IGF-I derives from that in the circulation.

In order to address this question, both immature and adult rats were subjected to UNX.[13] Remnant kidneys were removed after 24 and 48 hrs and compared to control kidneys, i.e., kidneys removed initially from the same animals. IGF-I gene expression in control (C) and remnant (R, compensated) kidneys was measured with total RNA using solution hybridization/RNase protection assays. As shown in Figure 3, steady-state levels of IGF-I mRNA were decreased in remnant kidneys compared with controls in adult rats. In contrast, IGF-I mRNA levels in remnant kidneys from immature rats were significantly increased (3-4 fold) compared with control kidneys. This increase in IGF-I mRNA was seen as early as 24 hrs following UNX and was confirmed by in situ hybridization. It appears, therefore, that in the developing or immature rat, local over-expression of IGF is central to the regeneration observed with UNX.

Differences in the regenerating capacity could also be due to altered sensitivity to growth factors. Binding of IGF-I and IGF-II to membranes prepared from remnant kidneys was slightly reduced as compared with controls in adult rats. In contrast, IGF-I and IGF-II binding to kidney membranes was increased in remnant kidneys from immature rats. The increase in IGF-II binding was significant in whole kidneys (20.5 ± 1.6 vs $15.5 \pm 0.5\%$ in remnant vs control, $p < 0.05$). IGF binding was not significantly increased in whole remnant kidneys from immature rats. However, when the cortex and medulla were dissected apart and IGF-I binding determined with membranes prepared separately, IGF-I binding to cortical membranes was significantly increased in remnant kidneys compared with controls (4.9 ± 0.6 vs $3.3 \pm 0.2\%$; $p < 0.05$). Medullary IGF-I binding was higher (9-10%) but did not differ between groups and could explain the lack of change seen in total kidney IGF-I binding in immature rats. To determine whether the increased IGF-I and IGF-II binding seen in remnant kidneys from immature rats was due to increased gene expression, steady state levels of IGF-I and IGF-II receptor mRNAs were measured using solution hybridization. Both IGF-I and IGF-II/M-6-P receptor mRNAs were significantly increased within 24 hrs of UNX in immature rats. In contrast, consistent with the binding data, receptor mRNA levels in adult rats were decreased.

In summary, there appear to be differential mechanisms initiating CRG following UNX during development. CRG in the adult animal is GH-dependent, since suppression of the elevated GH levels following injection of GRF-AN prevents hypertrophy. Furthermore, this effect of GH is probably not mediated by local IGF-I production. Whether the effect of GH on CRG in adult animals is a direct effect (via GH receptors, which are abundant in the kidney) or possibly via circulating IGF-I remains to be determined.

In contrast, in the immature rat, CRG is GH-independent and is associated with increased expression of the IGF-I gene as well as an increase in IGF-I and IGF-II/M-6-P receptors, both at the level of gene expression and binding. The increased renal IGF-I gene expression seems to be GH-independent and further supports the notion that extrahepatic tissue production of IGF-I is regulated by other factors in addition to GH. This locally produced IGF-I could then act in a paracrine fashion to initiate the increases in hemodynamics and hyperplastic growth.

LIVER REGENERATION FOLLOWING PARTIAL HEPATECTOMY

Regeneration of liver tissue has been studied in the rat following surgical removal of 75% of the liver.[14] This procedure results in growth of the liver, commencing within the first 24 hrs and reaching completion within 7 days. A number of growth factors have been

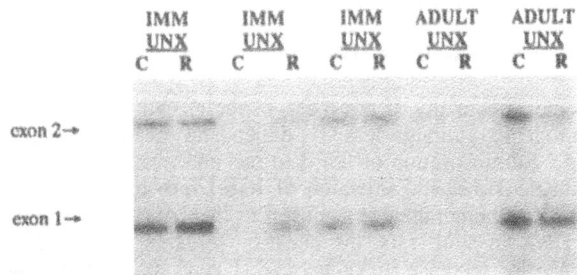

Figure 3. Measurement of IGF-I mRNA using a solution hybridization/RNase protection assay. Exons 1 and 2 lie upstream of exons encoding the mature peptide and are found in IGF-I mRNA variants. Renal IGF-I from immature and adult rats following unx in control (C) and remnant (R) kidneys.

proposed to be involved in the regeneration process and these include epidermal growth factor, transforming growth factor alpha, hepatocyte growth factor alpha, hepatopoietin B, acidic fibroblast growth factor and hepatic stimulatory substance.[14-16]

To prevent overcompensation, a number of inhibitory factors are also expressed, thereby attenuating the regenerative process, usually towards the latter part of the process. These include transforming growth factor beta, interleukin-1 beta, and hepatocyte proliferation inhibitor.[17-19]

To investigate the possible role of the IGF system in the process of liver regeneration, 50-day-old rats underwent partial (75%) hepatectomy. Control animals underwent sham operations. At various time intervals following surgery, animals were sacrificed and the livers removed. Regenerating livers were compared to control liver which includes the portions of the liver removed at the time of hepatectomy as well as livers removed from sham- operated controls.[20]

Using solution hybridization/RNase protection assays we measured expression of the IGF-I and IGF-II genes as well as the IGF-I receptor and the IGF-II/M-6-P receptor genes. No differences in expression were seen in the IGF-I, IGF-II or the IGF-I receptor genes when regenerating livers were compared with both types of control livers. In marked contrast, the steady-state levels of IGF-II/M-6-P receptor mRNA were increased in regenerating liver when compared with livers removed from the same animals or with sham-operated controls whose livers were removed at the same time points as those used for the regenerating livers. This significant increase in steady-state levels of mRNA was seen within the first 24 hrs following hepatectomy (Figure 4). Within a few days, the levels began falling and, by the end of the study period, mRNA levels were actually lower than control levels, suggesting that inhibitory factors come into play at this stage to prevent overcompensation. The changes in mRNA levels were associated with increased receptor protein. Specific IGF-II binding to liver membranes was increased in regenerating livers when compared to controls, and this effect was evident by 48 hrs. Furthermore, Western blot analysis with a specific antibody directed towards the IGF-II/M-6-P receptor demonstrated that this increased IGF-II binding was indeed due to increased levels of IGF-II/M-6-P receptor protein (Figure 5). Similar results were obtained by Baxter et al.[21]

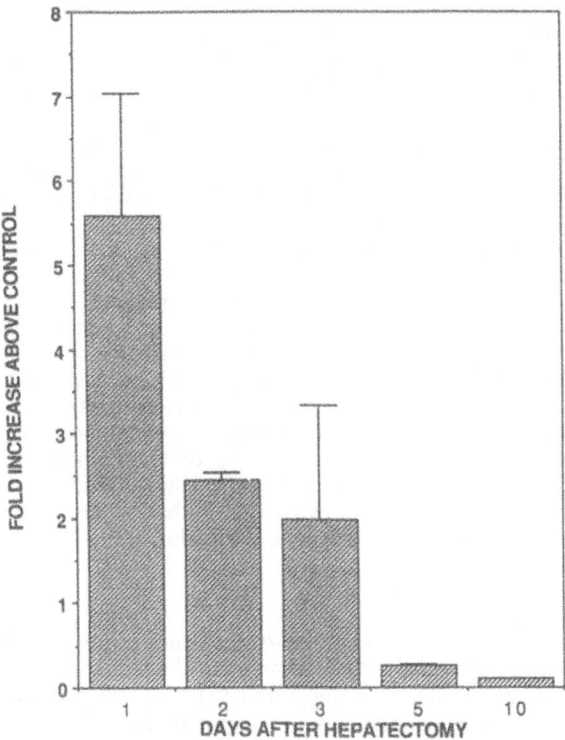

Figure 4. Steady state levels of IGF-II receptor mRNA were measured using a solution hybridization/RNase protection assay and quantitated by densitometric evaluation of the autoradiographs.

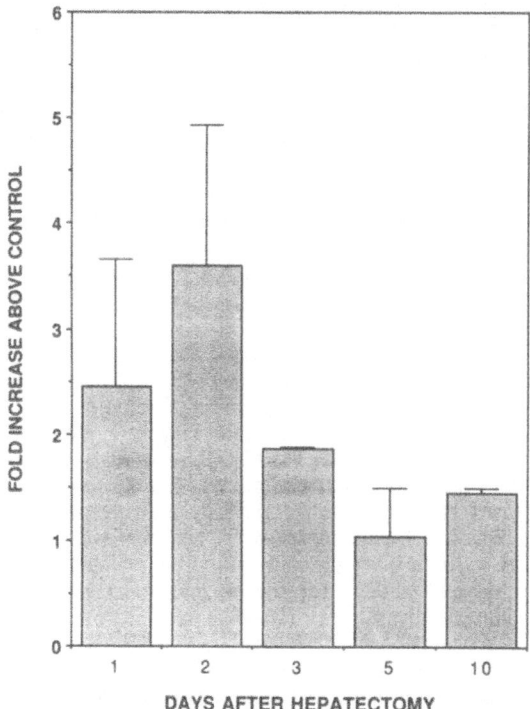

Figure 5. Western Blot analysis of the IGF-II receptor protein using a specific antibody. Quantitation was achieved by densometric analysis of autoradiographics.

Thus, liver regeneration in the rat is associated with increased levels of several components of the IGF system, specifically the IGF-II/M-6-P receptor and at least one of the characterized IGF-binding proteins (IGF-BP 1).[22] The IGF-II/M6-P receptor was originally thought not to transmit transmembrane signals due to its very short cytoplasmic tail and lack of tyrosine kinase activity. Indeed, its main function was considered to be internalization of hydrolases and IGF-II peptides, thereby directing these molecules to lysosomal compartments. The recent evidence that the IGF-II/M-6-P receptor can signal via a pertussis toxin - inhibitable G protein (probably G_i) has shed new light on its possible role in cellular function. Thus, one may speculate that the increased expression in liver regeneration may be important either to transmit some important signal involved in this process or, alternatively, it may be involved in the remodelling process by internalizing extracellular hydrolases. Since local production of IGF-I and IGF-II was not increased, it is possible that the stimulus for IGF-II/M-6-P receptor expression is derived from the circulation.

What role does the increased IGF-BP1 play in this process? Again, one can only speculate. Since the IGF-BPs have been shown to affect the biological actions of the IGFs, the increased liver production of IGF-BP1 may play a role in modulating the regenerative process. IGF-BP1 could potentiate the effects of the IGFs thereby enhancing the regeneration process or alternatively since it may also inhibit the action of IGFs, it could be a modulator of the regenerative process. Obviously, further studies using systemic infusions of IGFs and/or the binding proteins will help to clarify this situation.

Nerve And Muscle Degeneration

Numerous studies by Hansson et al. have established a role for IGF-I action in other regenerative and repair processes. After crushing of the sciatic nerve, there is a transient appearance of IGF-I immunoactivity in supporting Schwann cells.[23] The peak concentration of this presumably local production of IGF-I corresponded to the time at which cellular repair processes occur subsequent to initial inflammation. Similarly, autonomic or peripheral nerve trauma, regardless of mechanism, induces IGF-I immunoreactivity in Schwann cells as well as in associated fibroblasts of various types.[24-26]

Increased blood flow or pressure results in the appearance of IGF-I immunoreactivity, particularly in vascular smooth muscle cells.[27] Following denudation of arterial endothelium, high levels of IGF-I immunoreactivity are seen in invading endothelial cells and subsequently in the smooth muscle cells which comprise the neointima.[28] Other cell types which exhibit increased IGF-I immunoreactivity after injury include premyoblastic satellite cells in skeletal muscle,[29] connective tissue fibroblasts, skin epidermal cells and nasal mucosal epithelium. These numerous observations provide firm support for the hypothesis that IGF-I is intimately involved in numerous repair and regenerative processes in a wide variety of cell types.

CONCLUSIONS

In this review we have examined several examples of tissue regeneration where the process is associated with increased expression of the genes encoding various components of the IGF system - peptides, binding proteins and receptors. Indeed, the role of these elements in this process, though not yet proven, seems extremely likely. With the availability of recombinant DNA technology, not only is the measurement of gene expression more easily determined (as shown by the present studies) but, in addition, recombinant proteins are becoming available in large amounts. This will enable investigators to test the role of the IGF peptides and the binding proteins in diverse disease processes, including tissue regeneration. Finally, the findings in the studies presented in this review, though limited in scope, are potentially extrapolatable to many other organs (e.g., the pancreas) where regeneration is both desirable and clinically relevant.

REFERENCES

1. M. M. Rechler and S. P. Nissley, The nature and regulation of the receptors for insulin-like growth factors, Annu. Rev. Physiol. 47:425-42 (1985).
2. W. H. Daughaday and P. Rotwein, Insulin-like growth factors I and II. Peptide, messenger ribonucleic acid and gene structures, serum, and tissue concentrations, Endocr Rev. 10:68-91 (1989).
3. D. LeRoith, Insulin-like growth factors, in: "Molecular and Cellular Aspects," CRC Press, Boca Raton, Florida (1991).
4. I. Nishimoto, Y. Murayama, T. Katadi, M. Ui, and E. Ogata, Possible direct linkage of insulin-like growth factor I receptor and guanine nucleotide-binding proteins, J Biol Chem. 264:14029-38 (1989).
5. D.R. Clemmons, Insulin-like growth factor binding proteins, Trends in Endocr and Metab. 1:412-18 (1991).
6. H. A. Johnson and J. M. Vera-Rome, Compensatory renal enlargement: Hypertrophy vs. hyperplasia, Am J Pathol. 49:1-13 (1979).
7. S. E. Dicker, A. Greenbaum and C. A. Morris, Compensatory renal hypertrophy in hypophysectomized rats, J Physiol. 273:241-53 (1977).
8. A. Haramati, M.D. Lumpkin and S.E. Mulroney, Early rise in pulsatile growth hormone levels following unilateral nephrectomy in adult rats, (submitted).
9. S. E. Mulroney, M. D. Lumpkin and A. Haramati, Antagonist to GH-releasing factor inhibits growth and renal phosphate reabsorption in immature rats, Am J Physiol. 257:F29-F34 (1989).
10. M. D. Lumpkin, S. E. Mulroney and A. Haramati, Inhibition of pulsatile growth hormone secretion and somatic growth in immature rats with a synthetic GH-releasing factor antagonist, Endocrinology. 124(3):1154-59 (1989).
11. H. P. Guler, K. U. Eckard, J. Zapf, C. Bauer and E. R. Froesch, Insulin-like growth factor I increases glomerular filtration rate and renal plasma flow in man, Acta Endocrinol. 121:101-06 (1989).
12. H. P. Guler, J. Zapf, E. Scheiwiller and E. R. Froesch, Recombinant human insulin-like growth factor I stimulates growth and has distinct effects on organ size in hypophysectomized rats, Proc Natl Acad Sci USA. 85:4889-93 (1988).
13. S. E. Mulroney, H. Haramati, C. T. Roberts Jr. and D. LeRoith, Renal IGF-I mRNA levels are enhanced following unilateral nephrectomy in immature but not adult rats, Endocrinology. 128(5):2660-62 (1991).
14. G. K. Michalopoulos, Liver regeneration: molecular mechanisms of growth control, FASEB J. 4:176-87 (1990).
15. S. E. Raper, S. L. Burwen, M. E. Barker and A. L. Jones, Translocation of epidermal growth factor to the hepatocyte nucleus during rat liver regeneration, Gastroenterology. 92:1243-50 (1987).
16. J. E. Mead and N. Fausto, Transforming growth factor TGF-alpha may be a physiological regulator of liver regeneration by means of an autocrine mechanism, Proc Natl Acad Sci USA. 86:1558-62 (1989).

17. L. Braun, J.E. Mead, M. Panzica, R. Mikumo, G.I. Bell, and N. Fausto, Transforming growth factor-β mRNA increases during liver regeneration, Proc Natl Acad Sci USA. 85:1539-43 (1988).
18. T. Nakamura, R. Arakaki and A. Ichihara, Interleukin-1 is a potent growth inhibitor of adult rat hepatocytes in primary culture, Exp Cell Res. 179:488-97 (1988).
19. A. C. Huggett, H. C. Krutzsch and S. S. Thorgeirsson, Characterization of a hepatic proliferation inhibitor (HPI): effect of HPI on the growth of normal liver cells - comparison with transforming growth factor beta, J Cell Biochem. 35:305-14, 1987.
20. B. Burguera, H. Werner, M. Sklar, Z. Shen-Orr, B. Stannard, C. T. Roberts, Jr., S. P. Nissley, S. J. Vore, J. F. Caro and D. LeRoith, Liver regeneration is associated with increased expression of the insulin-like growth factor-II/mannose-6- phosphate receptor, Mol Endocrinol. 4:1539-45 (1990).
21. C. D. Scott and R. C. Baxter, Insulin-like growth factor- II/mannose-6-phosphate receptors are increased in hepatocytes from regenerating rat liver, Endocrinology. 126:2543-49 (1990).
22. K. L. Mohn, A. E. Melby, D. S. Tewari, T. M. Laz and R. Taub, The gene encoding rat insulin-like growth factor-binding protein 1 is rapidly and highly induced in regenerating liver, Mol Cell Biol. 11:1393-1401 (1991).
23. H-A. Hansson, B. Rozell and A. Skottner, Rapid axoplasmic transport of insulin-like growth factor I in the sciatic nerve of adult rats, Cell Tissue Res. 247:241-47 (1987).
24. H-A. Hansson, L. B. Dahlin, N. Danielsen, Evidence indicating trophic importance of IGF-I in regenerating peripheral nerves, Acta Physiol. Scand. 126:609-14 (1986).
25. H-A. Hansson, L. B. Dahlin, B. Lowenadler, Transient increase in insulin-like growth factor I immunoreactivity in rat peripheral nerves exposed to vibrations, Acta Physiol Scand. 132:35-41 (1988).
26. A. K. Nachemson, H-A. Hansson and G. Lundborg, Neurotropism in nerve regeneration: an immunohistochemical study, Acta Physiol Scand. 133:139-48 (1988).
27. H-A. Hansson, E. Jennische and A. Skottner, IGF-I expression in blood vessels varies with vascular load, Acta Physiol Scand. 129:165-69 (1987).
28. H-A. Hansson, E. Jennische and A. Skottner, Regenerating endothelial cells express insulin-like growth factor-I immunoreactivity after arterial injury, Cell Tissue Res. 250:499-505 (1987).
29. D. Edwall, M. Schallin, E. Jennische and G. Norstedt, Induction of IGF-I messenger RNA during regeneration of rat skeletal muscle, Endocrinology. 124:820-25 (1989).

DISCUSSION

C. Newgard: Among the genes that are activated in liver regeneration are albumin, PEPCK and a host of other genes that would be difficult to relate to growth promotion and proliferation. Is there any direct evidence that IGF-2 administration has any effects on the rate of liver regeneration?

D. LeRoith: Well, I don't think that anybody has tested that, because as you know, in the old days people used to study insulin and glucagon and there was a suggestion that perhaps insulin had some role on liver regeneration. I'm wondering whether their data perhaps relates to a secondary effect of some of the hormones that are involved. But the answer is that I don't think anybody has studied the direct effect of IGF-1 or IGF-2. I should mention a study by one group looking at the IGF-2 receptor in the liver at the recent endocrine meeting this last week showing that hypophysectomy and thyroidectomy actually affected the IGF-2 receptor. So again, what I'm saying is that I don't know the answer to this, but it is possible that some of those hormones like growth hormone, etcetera, may also be regulating these receptors in the regenerating situation. But nobody's yet tested specifically the role of any of these. Perhaps, the way to do it is by an elimination experiment using an antibody in a culture type system. But that hasn't been done. The problem, of course, of infusing something into the whole animal to determine regeneration may be difficult. However, I do think we have the tools to look at these sort of questions.

A. Vinik: Derek, you have an interesting model in terms of IGF. In the one situation with hyperplasia, there is an increase in the cell number and in the other situation with hypertrophy where you have an increase in cell size, you don't see the involvement of IGF. If you do a nephrectomy and you devise a means of inhibiting cell division, do you see the increase in the message?

D. LeRoith: The answer is that we have not tried to do it, but it's a very good idea. Obviously what you are suggesting -and what we are suggesting from this is that the growth hormone is involved in cell hypertrophy, and IGF's in the cell hyperplasia. It's known for example, that growth hormone can increase kidney size and IGF-1 can also increase the kidney size in early diabetic nephropathy where you get an increased glomerular filtration rate and plasma flow. It's possible that growth hormone is having one type of cellular effect, whereas IGF-1 is having a cell-division type of effect and both result in large kidneys. I cannot say what is the next step, but down the line that's what we would like to find out when we can devise the appropriate experiment.

N. Sarvetnick: I'd like to follow up and question the roles of some alternative hormones in the regulation of the IGF's and ask what kidney-related hormone would be a likely candidate growth regulator. How about vasopressin? Is it possible that a kidney-related factor may also be the hepatic growth factor?

D. LeRoith: I'd hate to speculate on vasopressin because I've never even thought it, but, I would suspect that in many of these situations there may be circulating hormones that are going to be involved, or that are going to change some other local factor. But I would be surprised, and I would speculate that every organ, perhaps, has it's own type of local regulatatory system. We know, for example, that in the kidney one of the strongest stimuli to IGF-1 production is erythropoietin. The corollary is also true. We know that if IGF-1 is given to an erythropoietin-type system one can actually stimulate erythropoietin production. In bone it differs; parathyroid hormone and estrogen affect IGF-1. In the ovary, FSH is involved with IGF-1 and IGF-1 receptor in steroidogenesis. So I would prefer for my own peace of mind to keep each thing compartmentalized, and I would hypothesize that each organ is going to have it's own specific factor. Now there are a number of growth factors - many of which we know and many that we don't know - which are obviously involved in this as well. The TGF alpha-beta family for example, the EGF's and so forth. I think that each system may use it's own group of factors. What the major stimulus is going to be, I don't know, but what the players in the field think is that it's going to be compartmentalized. Of course, you are going to have certain differences in opinion, but I'm just speculating, because that is what you asked me to do.

J. Nielsen: Isn't it true that someone has shown that there is a marked increase in growth hormone production with kidney and liver regeneration.

D. LeRoith: Has that been published? I don't remember having seen such a publication, but that doesn't mean I couldn't have seen and forgotten it.

THE EFFECTS OF IGF-I AND IGF-II ON CELL GROWTH AND DIFFERENTIATION IN THE CENTRAL NERVOUS SYSTEM

Thomas J. Lauterio, Ph.D.[1,2]
Eastern Virginia Medical School

[1]Eastern Virginia Medical School
  Departments of Internal Medicine and Physiology
  Norfolk, Virginia 23501

[2]Eastern Virginia Medical School
  Department of Veterans Affairs Medical Center
  Hampton, Virginia 23667

INTRODUCTION

The role of growth factors in central nervous system (CNS) function has been the focus of much research within the last decade. While much of the attention centered around nerve growth factor initially, other growth factors have also been shown to have a potential role in nervous system function. Among the most intriguing of these are the insulin-like growth factors I and II (IGF-I and IGF-II). As early as 1941, a report was published in which crude pituitary extracts were shown to increase the brain size of tadpoles.[1] Later studies following up on this initial observation demonstrated that the trophic factor involved in this response was growth hormone (GH) dependent[2] and that the factor causing the increased growth was IGF-I.[3]

The role of IGFs in the central nervous system is still far from resolved. Major questions regarding their function have not yet been addressed, such as whether both IGF-I and IGF-II exert effects via the type I or type II receptor, which cells respond to which factors and how IGF action in the CNS is mediated. Localization studies of the IGFs, their receptors and binding proteins have been undertaken, however, and may provide some insight to function.

LOCALIZATION OF IGF IN THE CNS

Both IGF-I and IGF-II peptides have been localized to specific brain regions, although sites for synthesis have not been well defined. It is possible that IGFs in the brain are transported from the periphery across the blood brain barrier or else gain entry through regions where this barrier is incomplete. Brain microvasculature does contain receptors for both IGFs and thus their active uptake into the brain is possible.[4,5] Brain access through the circumventricular organs has been well studied with regard to insulin,[6] and it is likely that IGFs could follow the same route into the brain due to their structural similarity with insulin and the overlap in receptor recognition. The synthesis of IGFs in the central nervous system has been reported by a number of investigators with discrepant results. Various laboratories have reported IGF-I and II mRNA to be present in the brain of adult and fetal rats,[7-9] but these researchers differ as to the regions of synthesis and cell types responsible for synthesizing the growth factors. Rotwein et al found IGF-I mRNA concentrated in the olfactory bulb and in the cervical-thoracic spinal cord,[9] but levels in the CNS were lower overall than those of IGF-II. The pons-medulla, cerebellum and hippocampus regions were rich in IGF-II mRNA in addition to the olfactory and cord areas. While *in situ* hybridization studies limit the regions of IGF-II synthesis to the leptomeninges and choroid plexus,[10] other investigators have found IGF-II mRNA in tissues other than these.[11] The discrepancy may be due to the techniques used by the groups since solution hybridization employed in the latter study is several fold more sensitive than *in situ* hybridization. Rotwein et al also determined which cell types synthesize IGFs. Using plating conditions to preferentially optimize survival of neurons versus glia, primary cultures were established from brains of 17 day old embryos.[9] IGF-I message was present in both neuron and glial cells, whereas IGF-II message was observed in only glial cell cultures.

Romanus and colleagues have demonstrated that the IGF-II mRNA present in the brain is also translated and processed into pre-pro-IGF-II which lends support to the notion that the IGF-II present in the CNS is synthesized there.[12] Brain concentrations of IGF-II peptide are much greater than those of IGF-I, and the distribution of IGF-II within the CNS varies considerably in specific regions[9] whereas that of IGF-I is more homogeneous. Even within the hypothalamus, a 10 fold concentration difference has been observed for IGF-II. Major questions remain as to what the predominant forms of IGFs are within the CNS. Haselbacher and Humbel[13] reported that a variant of IGF-II (big IGF-II) is present in amounts nearly equal to IGF-II in cerebrospinal fluid, whereas in other tissues, big IGF-II constitutes only a small fraction of the total IGF-II present. Sara[14] suggests that the major bioactive form of IGF-I for neural tissue is the truncated IGF-I whose cleavage product has been shown to bind the N-methyl-D-aspartate (NMDA) receptor. Thus, the predominant CNS products may be considerably different in structure as well as function from the peripheral species of these peptides.

IGF RECEPTORS IN THE CNS

In order for IGFs to exert effects in the CNS, the receptors for these factors need to be present in addition to the peptide. Numerous investigators have characterized IGF receptors in the brain and have found two species to exist.[15,16] The type II receptor is very similar to that found in the periphery, while the type I receptor has nearly the same affinity for both IGF-I and IGF-II. This "brain-type" IGF-I receptor is present in neuronal cells but the receptors found on glia are of the "peripheral" type.[17]

FUNCTION OF IGF IN THE CNS

Having established that IGFs and their receptors are present in the CNS, one turns to the question of function. In the periphery, IGFs have been shown to promote cell growth in multiple tissue types.[18-20] (See also Leroith et al in this volume) A similar function for IGFs has been proposed for the CNS. Studies in primary cells and cell lines strongly support this hypothesis. The survival of cultured chick dorsal root ganglionic (DRG) sensory neurons is greatly enhanced by the addition of rat IGF-II (multiplication stimulating activity or MSA) to the medium.[21] While initial studies suggested that neuron survival was dependent on NGF alone, this dependency theory has not held true for a number of models including the chick DRG. Recio-Pinto et al[22] confirmed the findings of Bothwell and extended them to chick sympathetic neurons. More recently, Svrzic and Schubert have demonstrated a survival function for IGF-I for chick embryonic cortical neurons.[23] In addition to promoting survival, IGFs also stimulate neurite outgrowth of these neurons. The percentage of neurons having neurites in the above study[21] was increased by MSA almost to the level achieved by nerve growth factor and at a 100 fold lower concentration than insulin suggesting that insulin effects on nervous tissue are mediated through the type I IGF receptor. This theory has since been demonstrated for a number of systems. Regarding sympathetic neurons, IGF-II and insulin appeared to be equipotent at stimulating neurite outgrowth. However, there is evidence that these peptides affect different populations of neurons. Insulin, in combination with NGF does not further increase the neurite outgrowth observed for either insulin or NGF alone. It is possible, therefore, that the two factors are acting on the same subpopulation of cells (NGF sensitive). IGF-II and NGF act in an additive manner when combined in culture to increase neurite outgrowth.

The mitogenic effects of insulin-like growth factors has been established for both primary cells and transformed cell lines. Both neuronal and glial cells increase ^{3}H-thymidine uptake in response to IGF-I[24] at concentrations (10^{-9} M) lower than those required for insulin (10^{-7} M) to achieve the same effect. IGF-I also increases RNA synthesis in primary fetal neurons.[25] These findings suggest a role for IGF-I in the CNS as a neurotrophic agent. Further, the ability of IGF-I (truncated form) to potently stimulate growth of the cerebral cortex has been shown.[26] In this report, non-truncated IGF-I had no effect on the cortex grafts, while truncated IGF-I also had a moderate stimulatory effect on growth of spinal cord grafts. Neither form of IGF-I elicited a response in hippocampal tissue.

In addition to enhancing cell survival and promoting mitogenesis, a role for IGFs in cell differentiation has been proposed. The number and complexity of neuritic arbors are increased in primary hypothalamic neurons grown in monoculture when exposed to low levels of IGF-I.[25,27] Levels of protein kinase C and GAP-43, markers of neuronal differentiation,[28] are also increased in cultured cells exposed to IGF-I. These effects can be produced by insulin, but at concentrations 2-5 fold greater than those required for IGF-I, indicating again that insulin's effects are via IGF-I receptor binding and not through its own receptor. Similar to IGF-I, IGF-II is also capable of stimulating neurite formation in SH-SY5Y neuroblastoma cells at physiological concentrations.[29]

MECHANISM OF ACTION OF IGFs IN THE CNS

The mechanism by which growth factors elicit their response has also been characterized to some extent. A number of reports have shown that axonal and dendritic growth occurs, at least in part, by increasing the cytoskeletal components that provide the framework of the neuron. Microtubules, consisting of α and β subunits are among the major and most important of such components and their synthesis is a prerequisite for growth. NGF exerts its effects on cell growth, in part due to its actions on tubulin synthesis and stabilization of the microtubule structure.[30] Nanomolar concentrations of IGF-II and insulin both increase α and β tubulin formation by increasing tubulin synthesis in a response curve that closely parallels the effects these hormones have on differentiation. This increased tubulin synthesis is observed regardless of whether the cells have been maintained in serum-free or serum-containing medium, whereas nerve growth factor stimulation of tubulin synthesis is serum dependent. The effect of IGF-II on differentiation is specific as antiserum to NGF does not diminish the ability of IGF-II to increase tubulin mRNA. Moreover, the level of tubulin mRNA increases relative to poly-A RNA and actin mRNA is unaffected by IGF treatment.[31]

The growth-promoting properties of the IGFs have been investigated to determine what role these factors may play in the regeneration process of nerves. The impetus to study IGF regulation of nerve regeneration is increased by the fact that regeneration is impaired in insulin-deficient[32] or hypophysectomized[33] rats that are known to be deficient in circulating IGF-I.[33-35] Further, treatment of streptozotocin-diabetic rats with insulin restores the nerve's regenerative potential concurrent with increasing IGF-I levels.[36] Direct evidence for IGFs growth promoting role has since been obtained using the freeze-injured[33] or crush lesion sciatic nerve model.[37] In the latter study, IGF-I was effective in stimulating regeneration regardless of whether it was administered to the dorsal root ganglia or locally at the site of the crush lesion. The role of IGFs in peripheral nerve regeneration is further discussed by Le Beau in this volume.

Neurons are not the only cells in the CNS that respond to IGFs. Both IGF-I and IGF-II stimulate development and differentiation of oligodendrocytes in culture.[38,39] A two-fold proliferation of O-2A cells is induced by as little as 3.3 ng/ml IGF-I in culture medium. IGF-I is more potent than IGF-II in this action, and can take the place of insulin at concentrations several orders of magnitude lower, (over 5 µg/ml insulin is required for minimal effect). Incorporation of ^{35}S methionine into sulfolipids is enhanced as is the synthesis of marker enzymes (e.g., glycerol-3-phosphate dehydrogenase) by IGF-I at physiological levels in glial cultures.[40] IGF-I also increases myelin basic protein (MBP) expression in oligodendrocytes cultured in serum-free defined medium.[41] Proliferative effects by IGFs on progenitor cells and metabolic effects in differentiated cells are apparently mediated by the IGF-I receptor, although the IGF-II receptor is present. However, it is still not clear whether IGF-I and IGF-II share equally in the physiological regulation of CNS growth and metabolism or whether one has a more dominant role in CNS function *in vivo*. While IGF-I is more potent at eliciting some physiological responses, IGF-II is present in the brain at 40 times the concentration of IGF-I, and thus may be the more

Table 1. The effects of IGF-I and II and their receptors on CNS function. Factors and receptors having demonstrated effects (+), no effects (0), or undetermined effects (?) are listed for each model system shown.

CNS Model Used	Peptide		Receptor	
	IGF-I	IGF-II	IGF-I	IGF-II
Chick DRG sensory neuron				
Survival	+	+	+	+?
Neurite outgrowth	+	+	+	+?
Chick sympathetic neuron survival	+	+	+	?
Primary hypothalmic neurons				
DNA synthesis	+	?	+	?
RNA synthesis	+	+	+	?
Differentiation	+	?	+	?
SH-SY5Y Neuroblasts				
Differentiation	+	+	+	?
Growth	+	+	+	?
Tubulin synthesis + stabilization	+	+	+	0
Increase NGF binding + action	+	+	+	0
Rat sciatic nerve regeneration				
Freeze-injured	+	?	+	?
Crush lesion	+	?	+	?
Oligodendrocytes				
Proliferation of O-2A cells	+	+	+	0
Differentiation to oligoden	+	+	+	0
Myelin basic protein synthesis	+	+	+	0

biologically important hormone. A table comparing the known effects of IGFs in CNS tissue and cells and the receptors involved in these actions has been compiled (Table 1).

Determining the effects of the IGF peptides on neurons and glia, does not resolve the question of their effects *in vivo*. Both IGFs are synthesized by the glia, whereas only neurons produce IGF-II so the mode of action of these hormones on various cells in the CNS depends on which of the two peptides is exerting the effect. For example, both peptides are capable of autocrine stimulation for oligodendrocytes, but IGF-II could work only in a paracrine or endocrine fashion on neurons. An example of the latter relationships could be the effect of IGF-II on neuroblastoma NGF receptors. When SH-SY5Y cells are maintained in serum-free media, NGF receptor binding disappears.[42] IGF-II supplementation alone is sufficient to restore NGF receptor binding in these cells. It is possible, therefore, that oligodendrocyte derived IGF-II is acting in a similar manner in the brain. Future research should certainly focus on the physiological mechanisms whereby IGF's are capable of mitigating neuronal loss, stimulating neuronal growth and differentiation as well as supporting the action of other nerve growth factors.

SUMMARY

Both IGF-I and IGF-II peptides have been localized to specific brain regions. The distribution of IGF-I is homogeneous whereas IGF-II appears to be more local. Two species of IGF receptors are found in the CNS. The type II (m6P) is similar to that in the periphery, but the type I has nearly the same affinity for IGF-I and IGF-II. IGF-I has now been shown to provide cell growth and survival as well as stimulate neurite outgrowth. Dorsal root ganglia and sympathetic neurons are sensitive to IGF-II and the action may be additive with NGF. Cells other than neurites, such as oligodendrocytes respond to the IGFs as well as primary and transformed lines. The mechanism of action has not been resolved but IDG-II appears to act via G-protein coupled activation of protein kinase C. Interaction between various growth factors and the IGFs may be due to up or down-regulation of the receptor predicated by the non-homologous peptide.

REFERENCES

1. S. Zamenhof, Stimulation of the proliferation of neurons by growth hormone. I: experiments on tadpoles, Growth. 5:123-39 (1941).
2. V.R. Sara, L. Lazarus, M.C. Stuart, and T. King, Fetal brain growth: selective action by growth hormone, Science. 186:446-47 (1974).
3. V.R. Sara, C. Carlsson-Skwirut, C. Andersson, E. Hall, B. Sjogren, A. Holmgren, and H. Jornvall, Characterization of somatomedins from human brain: identification of a variant form of IGF-I, Proc Natl Acad Sci USA. 83:4904-07 (1986).
4. K.R. Duffy, W.M. Pardridge, and R.G. Rosenfeld, Human blood-brain barrier insulin-like growth factor receptor, Metabolism. 37:136-42 (1988).
5. R.G. Rosenfeld, H. Pham, B.T. Keller, R.T. Borchardt, and W.M. Pardridge, Demonstration and structural comparison of receptors for insulin-like growth factor -I and -II (IGF-I and -II) in brain and blood-brain barrier, Biochem Biophys Res Commun. 149:159-66 (1987).
6. M.W. Schwartz, A.J. Sipols, S.E. Kahn, D.P. Latteman, G.J. Taborsky, R.N. Bergman, S.C. Woods, and D. Porte, Jr., Kinetics and specificity of insulin uptake from plasma in cerebrospinal fluid, Am J Physiol. 259:E378-83 (1990).
7. P.K. Lund, B.M. Moats-Staats, M.A. Hynes, J.G. Simmons, M. Jansen, A.J. D'Ercole, and J.J. Van Wyk, Somatomedin-C/Insulin-like growth factor-I and Insulin-like growth factor-II mRNAs in rat fetal and adult tissues, J Biol Chem. 261:14539-44 (1986).
8. L.J. Murphy, G.I. Bell, and H.G. Friesen, Tissue distribution of insulin-like growth factor I and II messenger ribonucleic acid in the adult rat, Endocrinology. 120:1279-82 (1987).
9. P. Rotwein, S.K. Burgess, J.D. Milbrandt, and J.E. Krause, Differential expression of insulin-like growth factor genes in the central nervous system, Proc Natl Acad Sci USA. 85:265-69 (1988).
10. F. Stylianpoulou, J. Herbert, M.B. Soares, and A. Efstratiadis, Expression of the insulin-like growth factor II gene in the choroid plexus and the leptomeninges of the adult rat central nervous system, Proc Natl Acad Sci USA. 85:141-45 (1988).
11. T.J. Lauterio, P.F. Aravich, and P. Rotwein, Divergent effects of insulin on insulin-like growth factor-II gene expression in the rat hypothalamus, Endocrinology. 126:392-98 (1990).
12. J.A. Romanus, Y.W.H. Yang, S.O. Adams, A.N. Sofair, L.Y.H. Tseng, S.P. Nissley, and M.M. Rechler, Synthesis of insulin-like growth factor II (IGF-II) in fetal rat tissues: translation of IGF-II ribonucleic acid and processing of pre-pro-IGF-II, Endocrinology. 122:709-16 (1988).
13. G. Haselbacher and R. Humbel, Evidence for two species of insulin-like growth factor II (IGF-II and "Big IGF-II) in human spinal fluid, Endocrinology. 110:1822-24 (1982).
14. V.R. Sara and C. Carlsson-Skwirut, Insulin-like growth factors in the central nervous system: biosynthesis and biological role. in: "Growth Factors: From Genes To Clinical Applications", V.R. Sara, K. Hall, and H. Low, eds., Raven Press, New York (1990).
15. V.R. Sara, K. Hall, H. von Holtz, R. Humbel, B. Sjogren, and L. Wetterberg, Evidence for the presence of specific receptors for insulin-like growth factor I (IGF-1) and 2 (IGF-2) and insulin throughout the human brain, Neurosci Lett. 34:39-44 (1982).
16. S. Gammeltoft, G.K. Haselbacher, R.E. Humbel, M. Fehlmann, and E. Van Obberghen, Two types of receptor for insulin-like growth factors in mammalian brain, Embo J. 4:3407-12 (1985).

17. A. Ota, Z. Shen-Orr, C.T. Roberts Jr, and D. LeRoith, TPA-induced neurite formation in a neuroblastoma cell line (SH-SY5Y) is associated with increased IGF-I receptor mRNA and binding, Mol Brain Res. 6:69-76 (1989).

18. E.R. Froesch, C. Schmid, J. Schwander, and J. Zapf, Actions of insulin-like growth factors, Annu Rev Physiol. 47:443-68 (1985).

19. M.M. Rechler and S.P. Nissley, The nature and regulation of receptors for the insulin-like growth factors, Annu Rev Physiol. 47:427-42 (1985).

20. W.H. Daughaday and P. Rotwein, Insulin-like growth factors I and II. Peptide, messenger ribonucleic acid and gene structures, serum and tissue concentrations, Endocr Rev. 10:68-91 (1989).

21. M. Bothwell, Insulin and somatomedin MSA promote nerve growth factor-independent neurite formation by cultured chick dorsal root ganglionic sensory neurons, J Neurosci Res. 8:225-31 (1982).

22. E. Recio-Pinto, M.M. Rechler, and D.N. Ishii, Effects of insulin, insulin- like growth factor II and nerve growth factor on neurite formation and survival in cultured sympathetic and sensory neurons, J Neurosci. 6:1211-19 (1986).

23. D. Svrzic and D. Schubert, Insulin-like growth factor 1 supports embryonic nerve cell survival, Biochem Biophys Res Comm. 172:54-60 (1990).

24. J. Shemer, M.K. Raizada, B.A. Masters, A. Ota, and D. LeRoith, Insulin- like growth factor I receptors in neuronal and glial cells, J Biol Chem. 262:7693-99 (1986).

25. S.K. Burgess, S. Jacobs, P. Cuatrecasas, and N. Sahyoun, Characterization of a neuronal subtype of insulin-like growth factor I receptor, J Biol Chem. 262:1618-22 (1987).

26. L. Olson, Ayer-LeLievre, T. Ebendal, M. Eriksdotter-Nilsson, P. Ernfors, A. Henshen, B. Hoffer, M. Giacobini, P. Mouton, M. Palmer, H. Persson, V. Sara, I. Stromberg, and C. Wetmore, Grafts, growth factors and grafts that make growth factors. in: "Progress in Brain Research", Vol. 82, S.B. Dunnett and S.J. Richards, eds., Elsevier Science, New York, (1990).

27. R.J. Robbins, J. Rasmussen, F. Naftolin, and I. Torres-Aleman, Growth factors and the developmental neurobiology of the hypothalamus, Acta Paediatr Scand. 367(suppl):93-97 (1990).

28. S.K. Burgess, N. Sahyoun, S.G. Blanchard, H. LeVine, K-J. Chang, and P. Cuatrecasas, Phorbol ester receptors and protein kinase C in primary neuronal cultures: development and stimulation of endogenous phosphorylation, J Cell Biol. 102:312-19 (1986).

29. J.F. Mill, M.V. Chao, and D.N. Ishii, Insulin, insulin-like growth factor II, and nerve growth factor effects on tubulin mRNA levels and neurite formation, Proc Natl Acad Sci USA. 82:7126-30 (1985).

30. D.G. Drubin, S.C. Feinstein, E.M. Shooter, and M.W. Kirscner, Nerve growth factor -induced neurite outgrowth in PC12 cells involves the coordinate induction of microtubule assembly and assembly-promoting factors, J Cell Biol. 101:1799-1807 (1985).

31. P. Fernyhough, J.F. Mill, J.L. Roberts, and D.N. Ishii, Stabilization of tubulin mRNAs by insulin and insulin-like growth factor I during neurite formation, Mol Brain Res. 6:109-20 (1989).

32. M.A. Bisby, Axonal transport of labeled protein and regeneration rate in nerves of streptozotocin-diabetic rats, Exp Neurol. 69:74-84 (1980).

33. J. Sjorberg and M. Kanje, Insulin-like growth factor (IGF-I) as a stimulator of regeneration in the freeze-injured rat sciatic nerve, Brain Res. 485:102-08 (1989).

34. L.S. Phillips and H.S. Young, Nutrition and somatomedin. II. Serum somatomedin activity in streptozotocin-diabetic rats, Diabetes. 25:516-27 (1976).

35. M. Maes, J.M. Ketelslegers, and L.E. Underwood, Low plasma somatomedin-C in streptozotocin induced diabetes: correlation with changes in somatogenic and lactogenic liver binding sites, Diabetes. 32:1060-69 (1983).

36. P.A.R. Ekstrom, M. Kanje and A. Skottner, Nerve regeneration and serum levels of insulin-like growth factor-I in rats with streptozotocin-induced insulin deficiency, Brain Res. 496:141-47 (1989).

37. M. Kanje, A. Skottner, J. Sjoberg and G. Lundborg, Insulin-like growth factor I (IGF-I) stimulates regeneration of the rat sciatic nerve, Brain Res. 486:396-98 (1989).

38. F.A. McMorris, R.W. Furlanetto, R.L. Mozell, M.J. Carson, and D.W. Raible, D.W. Regulation of oligodendrocyte development by insulin-like growth factors and cyclic nucleotides, Ann N Y Acad Sci. 101-09 (1990).

39. F.A. McMorris and M. Dubois-Dalcq, Insulin-like growth factor I promotes cell proliferation and oligodendroglial commitment in rat glial progenitor cells developing in vitro, J Neurosci Res. 21:199-209 (1988).

40. R.H.M. van der Pal, J.W. Koper, L.M.G. van Golde, and M. Lopes-Cardozo, Effects of insulin and insulin-like growth factor (IGF-I) on oligodendrocyte-enriched glial cultures, J Neurosci Res. 19:483-90 (1988).

41. R.P. Saneto, K.G. Low, M.H. Melner, and J. de Vellis, Insulin/insulin-like growth factor I and other epigenetic modulators of myelin basic protein expression in isolated oligodendrocyte progenitor cells, J Neurosci Res. 21:210-19 (1988).

42. E. Recio-Pinto, F.F. Lang and D.N. Ishii, Insulin and insulin-like growth factor II permit nerve growth factor binding and neurite formation response in cultured human neuroblastoma cells, Proc Natl Acad Sci USA. 81:2562-66 (1984).

GROWTH FACTOR EXPRESSION IN NORMAL AND DIABETIC RATS DURING PERIPHERAL NERVE REGENERATION THROUGH SILICONE TUBES

Jean M. Le Beau, Ph.D.[1]

[1]Eastern Virginia Medical School
Diabetes Institutes
855 West Brambleton Ave.
Norfolk, VA 23510

INTRODUCTION

Peripheral nerve regeneration is a unique example of tissue repair when considered at the cellular level. Individual neurons must survive axotomy, restore lost cellular components and each newly formed axon must retrace an appropriate pathway to its original anatomical connection. In addition, other nonneuronal cells residing in the nerve such as the glial, vascular and connective tissue components must also re-establish their precise morphological and functional relationship with the nerve during regeneration. Thus, from a biological standpoint, nerve regeneration raises many fundamental questions regarding the general nature of cell motility, cell-cell recognition, cell survival, and cell dedifferentiation, proliferation and differentiation - to name a few. Since many of these cellular events depend on growth and trophic factors for their occurrence, an analysis of growth factor expression during nerve regeneration may provide insight not only into their role during nerve regeneration, but also during wound repair in other nonneuronal tissues where regeneration can occur.

The capacity of damaged peripheral nerves to regenerate in the presence of diabetes mellitus is of concern since chronic neuropathy and delayed wound healing complicate this disorder. The silicone tube model of regeneration allows investigation of the effects of a systemic metabolic disorder such as diabetes on nerve repair *in vivo*. In this model, the severed ends of a transected rat sciatic nerve are sutured into a 14 mm long silicone tube.[1] Under normal metabolic conditions, significant nerve growth and myelination occur across a 10 mm gap and a gradient of maturation is established as a function of time and distance across the gap following nerve transection.[2-4] In experimentally induced diabetes, nerve regeneration and remyelination across the 10 mm gap is markedly impaired.[5] The molecular basis of this impairment is at present unknown. The silicone tube model of regeneration is a powerful experimental tool which provides a means to study the molecular basis of peripheral nerve growth and myelination. Its use in the study of nerve regeneration under normal metabolic conditions will be described. A model is proposed for use as a bioassay system to determine the effects of experimentally induced diabetes on growth factor expression during nerve regeneration and remyelination.

SILICONE TUBE MODEL TO STUDY REGENERATION

Investigators working with the silicone tube model of regeneration typically use 200-250 g adult Sprague-Dawley female rats. Stable anesthesia is induced by intraperitoneal injection of a mixture of Rompun (8 mg/kg) and Ketastet (80 mg/kg). The sciatic nerve is exposed by an incision into the lateral aspect of the thigh. After identifying its course from the sciatic notch to the tibial-peroneal bifurcation, the nerve is transected at the mid-thigh level and a 2 mm segment removed. The proximal and distal stumps are then sutured into the opposite ends of a 14 mm long silicone tube (Mentor Corp., Goleta, California) with a 9.0 ethilon suture. The inner diameter is 1.2 mm allowing passive non-constrictive cuffing of the nerve stumps. The dissection and tube implantation is designed to leave a 10 mm gap between the proximal and distal stumps (Figure 1). After securing both ends of the nerve, the sciatic compartment is closed with suture and the skin is closed with wound clips. After recovering from anesthesia, nerve regeneration can be followed for 2 to 154 days following nerve transection and tube implantation.

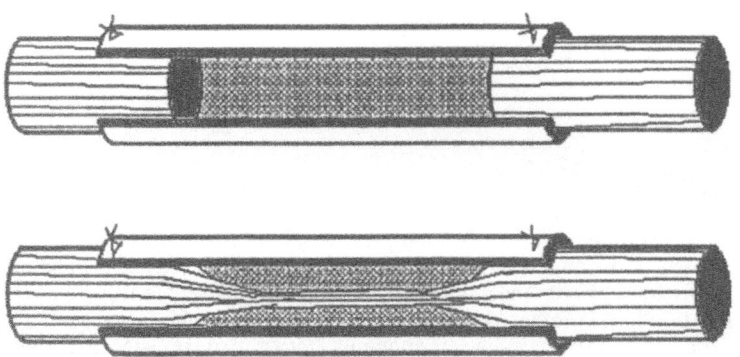

Figure 1. *Silicone tube model of regeneration.* (Top) Proximal and distal stumps of a rat transected sciatic nerve are sutured into opposite ends of a 14 mm long silicone tube. A 10 mm gap spans the severed nerve stumps. (Bottom) A new structure bridges the 10 mm gap by approximately 28 days following nerve transection and tube implantation. Electron microscopy reveals many newly regenerated and remyelinated axons.

At various times following nerve transection and tube implantation the regenerated nerve and associated tissues can be processed for morphological, biochemical or molecular studies. In addition, fluid which collects in the tube during regeneration can be extracted and examined for the presence of biological activity relevant to nerve regeneration. For morphological studies, the animal is deeply anesthetized and sacrificed by cardiac perfusion of phosphate buffered saline followed by continued perfusion with either a 2.5% glutaraldehyde - 1% paraformaldehyde solution (for electron microscopy studies) or 4% paraformaldehyde solution (for immunohistochemistry or in situ hybridization studies). Following fixation the regenerated nerve and tissues associated with its corresponding neurons (the L4 and L5 dorsal root ganglia and the area of spinal cord defined by the point of entry of spinal roots L4 and L5) are dissected free and further processed for the appropriate morphological studies.

For biochemical studies, the regenerated nerve and associated tissues (identified above) are carefully dissected free from anesthetized animals. Protein extracts are prepared from the tissue by homogenization in an ice-cold lysis buffer, followed by centrifugation. The precipitate is discarded and the supernatant is analyzed for protein concentration by Lowry's assay. The extracts can be stored indefinately at -70° C. Alternatively, the tissue can be removed and immediately extracted for RNA, and the RNAs analyzed by Northern blot analysis.

ADVANTAGES OF THIS MODEL AS A GROWTH ENHANCER AND EXPERIMENTAL TOOL

The silicone tube model of nerve regeneration has a number of advantages which make it an ideal tool for the study of nerve regeneration during normal and abnormal metabolic states. From a growth perspective, the silicone tube enhances nerve regeneration in several ways. First, the tube protects the nerve from the extraneural environment, thereby preventing contact with cells and other factors that may inhibit the regenerative response. Second, the silicone tube imposes a longitudinal orientation on regenerating fibers, minimizing the formation of a neuroma. Finally, the tube confines endogenous growth-promoting factors, that may be released during regeneration, to the nerve repair site.

From an experimental standpoint, the nerve regeneration model also has a number of unique features that highlight its importance as a basic science tool for examining nerve repair. First, the cellular events that occur during nerve regeneration can be precisely identified at the light and electron microscopic level as a function of both time following nerve transection, and placement along the 10 mm long proximal to distal axis of new nerve growth spanning the severed nerve stumps. Second, because the silicone tubes are non-porous and translucent, fluid that collects in the tube during regeneration can be harvested and assayed for protein content and identification of potential biological activity. Third, the regenerated nerve and associated tissues can be easily removed and tissue extracts can be prepared for immunoblotting and protein assay experiments to identify proteins important in the regenerative process. Finally, adjuncts that either potentially promote or inhibit nerve regeneration can be added to the silicone tube during nerve regeneration via an osmotic pump to evaluate their effects. Some of these applications will be illustrated in more detail as subsequent discussion focuses on investigations of normal peripheral nerve repair.

NERVE GROWTH AND MYELINATION DURING NERVE REGENERATION

When the severed ends of a rat sciatic nerve are sutured into a 14 mm long silicone tube, nerve growth and myelination occur in a reproducible manner across the 10 mm gap. The sequence of events have been described in both light and electron microscopic studies[2-4] and the occurrence and timing of the major cellular events are summarized in Table 1. Briefly, Schwann cell proliferation in the distal stump closely follows the transection of the nerve. Between 7 and 14 days, axons and Schwann cells appear to emerge together from the proximal stump, and advance towards the distal stump. At this time, blood vessel formation proceeds from both the proximal and distal stumps toward the mid-section of the tube. These events directly precede the onset of myelination which actively occurs between 14 and 21 days following tube implantation. By 21 days, thinly myelinated axons are found in the proximal region of the regenerated nerve. At later times, the 14 mm long tube is bridged by newly regenerated and remyelinated axons. Between 90 and 150 days following nerve transection, the growth of the nerve becomes markedly arrested.[6]

These studies demonstrate that the regeneration model has many features in common with peripheral nerve development including the events of nerve growth, myelination and node of Ranvier formation.[3,4] Since the morphological parameters of these cellular events are now well defined and easily identified as a function of both *time* following nerve transection and *space* along the proximal-distal axis of growth, the next step is to use the regeneration model to examine the expression of specific growth factor genes and proteins during nerve growth and myelination. What follows is a discussion of some of these studies and their potential relevance to the process of growth in general with emphasis on diabetic neuropathy.

Table 1. Sequence of cellular events during sciatic nerve regeneration through silicone tubes

Post-transectional Day	Event
0 - 7	Cell migration into tube from both stumps; Schwann cell proliferation in distal stump
7 - 14	Axon sprouting from proximal stump; vascular sprouting from both stumps
14 - 21	Onset of myelination in proximal stump
28 - 42	Regenerated axons bridge 10mm gap
90	Axons reach neuromuscular junction
154	Regenerated nerve stabilizes in growth

ROLE OF ENDOGENOUS DIFFUSIBLE FACTORS IN PERIPHERAL NERVE REGENERATION

Within hours of suturing the severed proximal and distal nerve stumps into the silicone tube, a clear serous fluid fills the entire tube.[7] This fluid continuously surrounds the regenerated nerve structure throughout the period of regeneration and can be sampled for the presence of endogenous neuronotrophic and neurite-promoting factors. Studies using the silicone tube model of regeneration have shown that neuronotrophic factors which enhance the survival of cultured neurons representing all three sciatic nerve components (sensory, sympathetic and motor) are present in the fluid during nerve regeneration.[7,8] Highest levels of the factors are present at a time when they could most influence neuronal survival and regeneration. Furthermore, fluid collected from these tubes during regeneration also contains neurite-promoting factors whose appearance corresponds with neurite outgrowth *in vivo*.[9]

Regeneration-promoting factors can operate directly on regenerating neurons as described above, or indirectly by initiating responses in Schwann cells. These cells are a critical constituent of the peripheral nerve. They are a source of trophic support for the neurons and their movement and proliferation are fundamental to the process of peripheral nerve regeneration and remyelination. It is conceivable therefore that soluble factors promoting these activities would be present in the fluid that accumulates in the silicone tubes during peripheral nerve regeneration. Regeneration-conditioned fluid (RCF) was aspirated from silicone tubes at various times during nerve regeneration and tested for biological activity in assays designed to measure Schwann cell migration and proliferation. Figure 2 shows the migration response of Schwann cells *in vitro* to RCF.[10] Schwann cells were placed into the upper compartment of a modified Boyden chamber, separated from the bottom well containing RCF by an 8-um pore size filter. Under these conditions, Schwann cells move through the pores and attach to the underside of the filter. The effect is dependent on the age of the fluid; RCF collected at 7 days following nerve transection had biological activity that was 87-fold greater than control fluid. The motility-promoting activity in RCF correlates well with the occurrence of Schwann cell movement *in vivo* in that Schwann cells do not appear to move out from the severed nerve stumps until about 3 days following nerve transection. Their movement then becomes continuous, occurring in tandem with the advancement of regenerated axons across the 10 mm gap.

The effect of RCF on Schwann cell proliferation was also examined by ^{3}H-thymidine incorporation into the DNA of purified Schwann cell cultures.[10] Figure 3 shows that RCF stimulated ^{3}H-thymidine incorporation to a significantly great extent than in the control, and the amount of stimulation was dependent upon the age of the fluid. The two peaks of

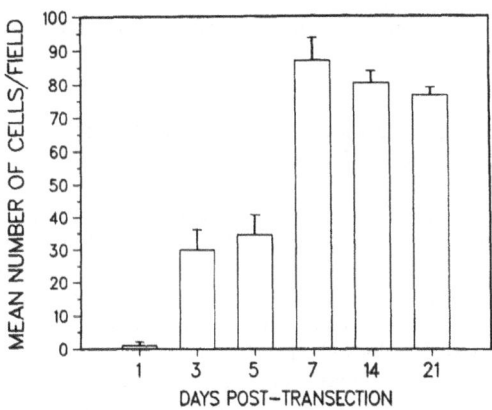

Figure 2. *Migration of Schwann cells to RCF*. Cells were incubated for 4 h at 37°C in the presence of RCF (540 ug of protein per well diluted in DMEM) collected at different post-transactional days. 3-6 assays were conducted with RCF collected from different nerves for each time point tested. Data are expressed as the mean number of cells per field that migrated through the filter plus the standard error of the mean. Schwann cells did not migrate in response to DMEM alone. (1) 1-day-old RCF; (3) 3-day-old RCF; (5) 5-day-old RCF; (7) 7-day-old RCF; (14) 14- day-old RCF; (21) 21-day-old RCF. [From Le Beau et al., Brain Res. 459:93 (1988). Reprinted with permission.]

biological activity characteristic of both 1-, 3- and 14-day-old fluid is consistent with the peaks of Schwann cell mitosis occurring *in vivo* during Wallerian degeneration and the onset of myelination respectively.

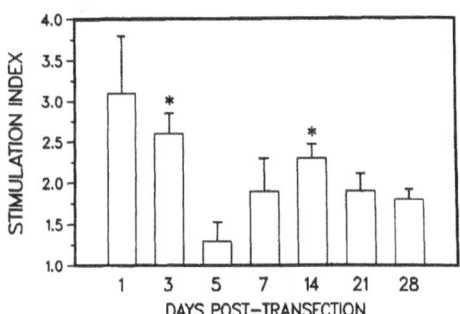

Figure 3. *Schwann cell mitogenic activity of RCF*. Schwann cells were incubated 72 h with RCF (108 ug of protein per well collected at different post-transactional days). ^{3}H-thymidine was added to the cultures and after 24 h incubation, the cells were fixed and harvested for scintillation counting. Each time point was assayed with RCF from at least three different nerves, and each nerve was assayed in quadruplicate. The data are expressed as the mean plus the standard error of the mean of stimulation indices (cpm in mitogen/cpm in control) per time point of RCF. The control (DMEM alone) value is equal to one. (*) Groups significantly different from control at $p \leq .05$ using Dunn's multiple comparison test. (1) 1-day-old RCF; (3) 3-day-old RCF; (5) 5-day-old RCF; (7) 7-day-old RCF; (14) 14-day-old RCF, (21) 21-day-old RCF. (28) 28-day-old RCF. [From Le Beau et al, Brain Res. 459:93 (1988). Reprinted with permission.]

In conclusion, these studies demonstrate that soluble neuronal- and Schwann cell-promoting factors are produced and released during peripheral nerve repair. The roles and identification of these endogenous growth factors may be further elucidated when specific antibodies and antagonists are successfully applied to nerve regeneration tubes. Identification and increased understanding of the nature of these factors should provide significant information on the role of diffusible trophic factors during nerve repair under both normal and abnormal conditions of regeneration. More importantly, the observation that these factors appear in the conditioned medium during normal nerve regeneration suggests that they may be potentially used to enhance regeneration-compromised states, such as diabetes.

ROLE OF INTRACELLULAR GROWTH FACTORS DURING NERVE REGENERATION THROUGH SILICONE TUBES

Another approach to examining growth factor expression during nerve regeneration is to focus on intracellular as opposed to extracellular events that may be important in mediating the growth and differentiation of cells. pp60[c-src] is a 60 kDA intracellular phosphoprotein which functions as a tyrosine kinase *in vitro*[11] and is associated with the plasma membrane of cells.[12] Thus, pp60[c-src] is ideal as a possible mediator of cell-cell interactions involved in nerve growth and myelination during regeneration. Since earlier studies had shown that pp60[c-src] was important in neuronal signaling and neurite outgrowth during development,[13,14] it was asked whether this protein was important in mediating nerve growth and myelination during regeneration through the silicone tubes.[15] To determine whether pp60[c-src] was a factor during peripheral nerve regeneration, sciatic nerve segments were extracted at various time points following nerve transection and tube implantation and analyzed by in vitro kinase assays. Figure 4a shows the expression of pp60[c-src] kinase

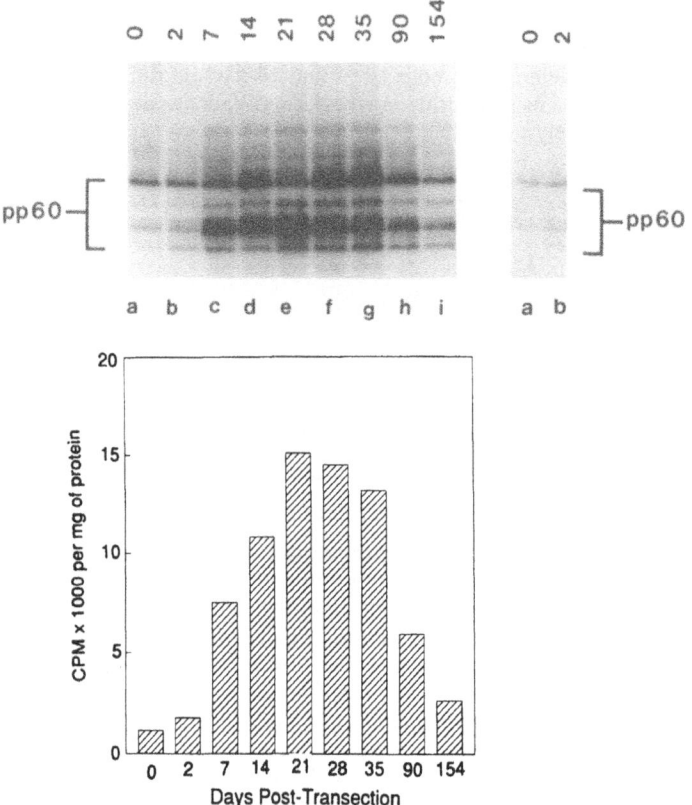

Figure 4. *Induction of pp60[c-src] kinase activity in regenerated nerve.* (A) *In vitro* kinase assays were carried out and analyzed by PAGE. Lanes: a, control sciatic nerve; b, 2 days post-transection (DPT); c, 7 DPT; d, 14 DPT; e, 21 DPT; f, 28 DPT; g, 35 DPT; h, 90 DPT; i, 154 DPT. (B) The bands corresponding to pp60[c-src] in (A) were excised from the gel and the ^{32}P-content was determined as a function of days following nerve transection. The kinase activity is expressed as counts per minute per milligram of total extract protein. Maximum induction of kinase activity was observed at 21 DPT. [From Le Beau et al. J Neurosci Res. 28:299 (1991). Reprinted with permission.]

activity in regenerated nerve segments as a function of time following nerve transection.[15] Minimal kinase activity was present in control sciatic nerve (lane a) and at 2 days following nerve transection (lane b). Kinase activity began to rise at 7 days post-nerve transection (lane c) coincident with the initiation of neurite outgrowth *in vivo*. This activity reached peak levels of activity between 21 and 35 days (lanes e-g) when the occurrence of neurite outgrowth and myelination are most vigorous, and decreased thereafter, approaching control levels by 154 days (lane i) when nerve growth arrests. Quantification of the protein bands by scintillation spectrometry is shown in Figure 4b.

The maximum kinase activity in nerves harvested at 21 days post-nerve transection was approximately 13-fold greater than control. Immunoblotting experiments confirmed that pp60^{c-src} is increased during regeneration, with the greatest enrichment confined to the middle regenerated segment where regenerated and remyelinated axons were most abundant. The least amount of protein was associated with the distal segment which had few if any regenerated axons. The increased kinase activity and protein expression of pp60^{c-src} in regenerated nerve coincided with the occurrence of axonal sprouting and remyelination *in vivo* suggesting that pp60^{c-src} may facilitate these events during regeneration.

The cells responsible for the increased c-src protein and respective kinase activity during nerve regeneration were determined by in situ hybridization. Figure 5 shows the localization of c-src mRNA during regeneration.[15] mRNA was present at significant levels in regenerated nerve segments (c and d) at 28 days post-nerve transection as compared to tissue treated with sense probe (a and b). The message appeared to be associated with Schwann cells which constitute the major cell bodies in the regenerated nerve. C-src mRNA was also detected in the sensory and motor neurons innervating the regenerated sciatic nerve (g,h, k and l) at levels significantly greater than corresponding tissue hybridized with sense probe (e,f, i and j).

This latter finding suggests that pp60^{c-src} is also synthesized in neuronal cell bodies and axonally transported to repair sites during regeneration. A further understanding of the role of the second messenger system in nerve regeneration will undoubtedly contribute to new approaches regarding the facilitation of nerve growth.

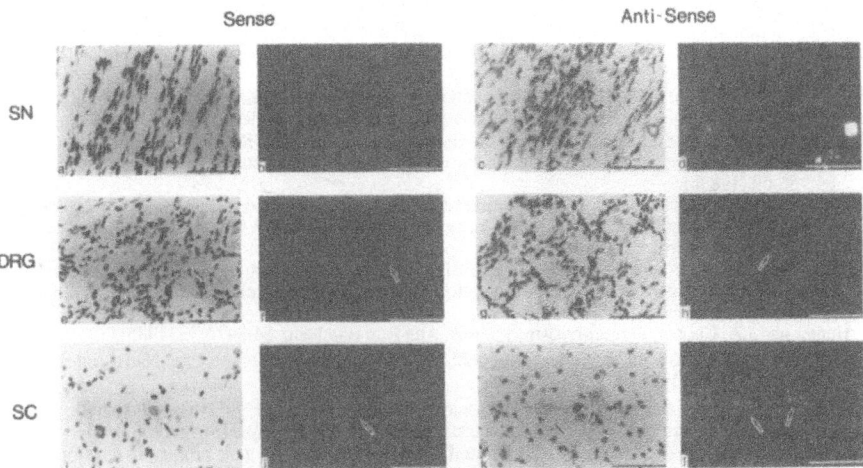

Sense   Anti-Sense

SN

DRG

SC

Figure 5. *Localization of c-src-specific mRNA by in situ hybridization on regenerated tissues.* Cryostat sections from regenerated tissue were hybridized with sense (a,b,e,f,i,j) and anti-sense (c,d,g,h,k,l) single stranded c-*src* RNA probes. **a, b,** Bright- and filtered-field photograph of a longitudinal section of regenerated nerve processed at 28 days post-transection with the sense strand probe. **c, d,** Bright- and filtered-field photograph of a longitudinal section of regenerated nerve processed at 28 days post-transection with the anti-sense strand probe. **e, f,** Bright- and filtered-field photograph of a longitudinal section of dorsal root ganglia processed at 28 days post-transection with the sense strand probe. Arrows point to sensory neurons. **g, h,** Bright- and filtered-field photograph of a longitudinal section of dorsal root ganglia processed at 28 days post-transection with the anti-sense strand probe. Arrows point to sensory neurons. **i, j,** Bright- and filtered-field photograph of a transverse section of spinal cord processed at 28 days post-transection with the sense strand probe. Arrows point to motor neurons. **k, l,** Bright- and filtered-field photograph of a transverse section of spinal cord processed at 28 days post-transection with the anti-sense strand probe. Arrows point to motor neurons. All bars represent 100 μm. [From Le Beau et al, J Neuro Sci Res. 28:299 (1991). Reprinted with permission.]

SUMMARY

The silicone tube model of regeneration has proved to be an invaluable tool for experimental studies aimed at understanding expression of growth factors during normal and abnormal metabolic states of regeneration. Since the morphological parameters of nerve growth and myelination are well-defined and easily identified in this model, the expression of both diffusible and intracellular-acting growth factors can be readily correlated with the occurrence of these cellular events. These studies facilitate the study of the cellular and molecular events that accompany regeneration. Further, because the sciatic nerve can be traced up to its corresponding neurons, growth factor gene expression can also be studied by in situ hybridization and Northern blotting techniques. This is particularly important in defining the cell source of extracellularly released growth factors. Finally, and most importantly, the regeneration process in the normal or diseased metabolic state (such as diabetes) can be manipulated via the administration of adjuncts to the tube that either promote or inhibit regeneration. Further studies in this regard, and in the identification of growth factors involved and their role during regeneration should shed some light on the pathogenesis and possible means of mitigating or reversing diabetic neuropathy.

REFERENCES

1. G. Lundborg, R.H. Gelberman, F.M. Longo, H.C. Powell, and S. Varon S, In vivo regeneration of cut nerves encased in silicone tubes: growth across a six-millimeter gap, J Neuropathol Exp Neurol. 4:412-22 (1982).
2. L.R. Williams, F.M. Longo, H.C. Powell, G. Lundborg, and S. Varon, Spatial-temporal progress of peripheral nerve regeneration within a silicone chamber: parameters for a bioassay, J Comp Neurol. 218:460-40 (1983).
3. J.M. Le Beau, H.C. Powell, and M.H. Ellisman, Node of Ranvier formation along fibres regenerating through silicone tube implants: a freeze-fracture and thin-section electron microscopic study, J Neurocytol. 16:347-58 (1987).
4. J.M. Le Beau, M.H. Ellisman, and H.C. Powell, Ultrastructural and morphometric analysis of long-term peripheral nerve regeneration through silicone tubes, J Neurocytol. 17:161-72 (1988a).
5. F.M. Longo, H.C. Powell, J.M. Le Beau, M.R. Gerrero, H.M. Heckman, and R.R. Myers, Delayed nerve regeneration in streptozotocin diabetic rats. Muscle Nerve. 9:385-93 (1986).
6. R.D. Fields, J.M. Le Beau, F.M. Longo, and M.H. Ellisman, Nerve regeneration through artificial tubular implants, Prog Neurobiol. 33:87-134 (1989).
7. F.M. Longo, M. Manthorpe, S.D. Skaper, G. Lundborg, and S. Varon, Neuronotrophic activities accumulate in vivo within silicone nerve regeneration chambers, Brain Res. 262:109-16 (1983a).
8. F.M. Longo, S.D. Skaper, M. Manthorpe, L.R. Williams, G. Lundborg, and S. Varon, Temporal changes in neuronotrophic activities accumulating in vivo within nerve regeneration chambers, Exp Neurol. 81:756-69 (1983b).
9. F.M. Longo, E.G. Hayman, G.E. Davis, E. Ruoslahti, E. Engvall, M. Manthorpe, and S. Varon, Neurite-promoting factors and extracellular matrix components accumulating in vivo within nerve regeneration chambers, Exp Neurol. 81:756 (1984).
10. J.M. Le Beau, M. LaCorbiere, H.C. Powell, M.H. Ellisman, and D. Schubert, Extracellular fluid conditioned during peripheral nerve regeneration stimulates Schwann cell adhesion, migration and proliferation, Brain Res. 459:93-104 (1988b).
11. T. Hunter and J.A. Cooper, Protein-tyrosine kinases, Ann Rev Biochem. 54:897-930 (1985).
12. S.A. Courtneidge and J.M. Bishop, Transit of pp60^{c-src} to the plasma membrane, Proc Natl Acad Sci USA. 78:7117-21 (1982).
13. C.G. Shores, M.E. Cox, and P.F. Maness, A tyrosine kinase related to pp60^{c-src} is associated with membranes of Electrophorus electricus electric organ, J Biol Chem. 262:9477-85 (1987).
14. P.F. Maness, M. Aubry, C.G. Shores, L. Frame, and K.H. Pfenninger, c-src gene product in developing rat brain is enriched in nerve growth cone membranes, Proc Natl Acad Sci USA. 85:5001-05, 1988.
15. J.M. Le Beau, B. Tedeschi, and G. Walter, Increased expression of pp60^{c-src} protein-tyrosine kinase during peripheral nerve regeneration, J Neurosci Res. 28:299-309 (1991).

ONCOGENES AND CELL GROWTH

Timothy J. Bos[1]

[1]Eastern Virginia Medical School
Department of Microbiology and Immunology
P.O. Box 1980
Norfolk, VA 23501

INTRODUCTION

Whether a cell enters a specific growth or differentiation program is governed in part by its response to signals from various external stimuli - such as polypeptide growth factors. The signals are transmitted through the cell to the nucleus where they can be turned into a response by the cell through activation of various genetic programs.

Much of our understanding of the mechanisms involved in the regulation of cell growth and tumorigenesis has come from the study of oncogenes and proto-oncogenes.

Clues to the functions that proto-oncogenes play in normal cell growth and differentiation have come from a number of important discoveries. A report in 1983 by Doolittle and co-workers[1] was a crucial landmark. It announced that the oncogene carried by simian sarcoma virus - sis - was identical to a growth factor secreted from platelets, called platelet-derived growth factor. This was the first instance in which a specific biological function could be found for the product of a known oncogene. In addition, it provided the first evidence that oncogenes might be involved in growth control. Since this discovery, computer-aided searches of the data bases have revealed a number of other interesting homologies between oncogenes and cellular genes. C-erb B was found to be the EGF receptor;[2] C-fms is the macrophage colony stimulating factor receptor.[3] C-erb A is identical to the thyroid hormone receptor[4] and c-Jun was found to be homologous to the yeast transcription factor GCN4,[5] and was later identified as a major component of the mammalian AP-1 transcription factor complex.[6] It has become clear that the products of proto-oncogenes play critical roles in the regulation of cell growth and differentiation and are not merely, as the name implies, cryptic cancer causing genes.

CLASSES OF ONCOGENES

There are two general classes of oncogenes and proto-oncogenes. The first class is referred to as dominant. The majority of oncogenes that have been characterized belong to this class. They are characterized by the fact that expression of a mutated gene product or overexpression of a normal gene product will lead to cell transformation. The second class is referred to as suppressor genes. The existence of suppressor genes is a relatively recent discovery.[7] Their existence was first hypothesized from experimental evidence in which fusion of a normal cell with a tumor cell would lead to loss of the tumor cell phenotype. Something in the normal cell was suppressing activity by the tumor cell. In addition, the *existence of a number of hereditary tumors associated with chromosome deletions, such as* retinoblastoma and Wilms' tumor, suggested the existence of suppressor genes. Suppressor genes - often called anti-oncogenes - are characterized by the fact that expression is required not to stimulate growth but to suppress cell growth, and that inactivation of a suppressor gene leads to cell transformation.

ONCOGENES AND CELL SIGNALLING

The products of oncogenes can be found at all levels in various signalling pathways (Table 1). In addition to growth factors, such as Sis and Int-2 and growth factor receptors, such as c-Erb B, c-Erb B - 2 and c-Fms, a number of oncogenes have been assigned functions as intracellular signalling molecules. These include the nonreceptor tyrosine kinases such as the Src family; GTP binding proteins such as the Ras family; and the cytoplasmic ser/thr kinases such as Mos and Raf. In addition to the signalling molecules, many proto-oncogenes have been identified as nuclear DNA binding proteins. Examples include Myc, Myb, Fos, Jun, Ets, Rel and Ski. This group of oncogenes act as effector molecules - turning incoming signals into a response by the cell - presumably, by activating specific genetic programs. In addition to these dominantly acting oncogenes, several

Table 1. Classification and Function of Cell-derived Proto-oncogene Products*

General Category	Proto-Oncogenes	Homology with known cellular genes
Growth Factors	sis int-2	B-chain of PDGF
Growth Factor Receptors	erb-B fms trk	EGF-receptor CSF-1 receptor NGF receptor
Membrane-associated non receptor tyrosine kinases	src yes lck fgr fps/fes	
GTP-binding proteins	H-ras K-ras N-ras	
Cytoplasmic ser/thr kinases	raf mos	
Nuclear DNA-binding proteins	c-myc N-myc L-myc c-myb c-jun c-fos c-rel c-ets c-ski c-erb A	Part of the AP-1 transcription factor NFKB-related thyroid hormone receptors

* This is a partial list of known Proto-oncogenes

suppressor oncogenes have been identified whose activity is thought to suppress cell growth rather than to stimulate it. These include RB, P53 and the Wilms' tumor gene.

ONCOGENIC ACTIVATION

In the normal cellular setting the products of proto-oncogenes are not oncogenic, in fact they play essential roles in controlling cell growth and differentiation. They are believed to become oncogenic when their activity within the cell is altered; resulting in a loss of normal control over function, activity or regulation.

There are several mechanisms by which proto-oncogenes can be activated to become oncogenic. The first method is by point mutation. The *ras* oncogene provides a classic example. The normal Ras protein is a GTP-binding protein. It normally exists in an inactive state bound to GDP. An incoming signal induces the Ras protein to bind GTP which puts it in an active state where it can now pass on the signal. Coupled with GTP binding activity is activation of GTPase activity that hydrolyzes GTP to GDP thus inactivating itself. Only a short signal pulse is sent through the Ras protein before it is inactivated. Ras can be oncogenically activated by point mutations in a single nucleotide which result in a single amino acid change. The most common mutation site is codon 12 in which a glycine is replaced by any other amino acid. Other hot spots for mutation are codons 13 and 61.[8] Interestingly these mutations abolish the GTPase activity of Ras thus keeping it in a continuously active state. Therefore a constitutive signal is sent from the Ras protein even in the absence of an incoming stimulus. This signal, telling the cell to divide, is no longer under cellular control and results in a continuous signal being transmitted to the nucleus. A variety of chemical carcinogens as well as UV and gamma irradiation can cause point mutations. Ras mutations are found in a large number of human cancers. The list includes adenocarcinoma of lung, colon and pancreas as well as some leukemias.

Another type of mutation commonly found are structural deletions. These are often associated with receptor proto-oncogenes. An example is the c-Erb B proto-oncogene better known as the epidermal growth factor receptor. Receptors have several functional domains. One is extracellular and is responsible for ligand binding - it has a specific affinity with a specific growth factor. The other is intracellular and usually has an enzymatic activity such as a kinase activity that is responsible for signal transduction to the next protein in the signal chain. In a normal cell, in the absence of ligand, the c-Erb B growth factor receptor contains an inactive kinase. Once ligand binds to the receptor, a conformational change occurs in which the intracellular kinase domain now becomes active. The active receptor sends a signal to the next protein in the signal chain. An oncogenic form of c-Erb B such as the viral Erb B protein, has deleted most of its extracellular domain and can no longer bind to epidermal growth factor (EGF).[9] It has however retained its intracellular kinase domain and this domain is in the active conformation. The truncated protein thus sends a constitutive signal in the absence of growth factor much like the point mutation in the ras proteins. This results in the cell being fooled into entry into a cell growth program.

Mutations are generally associated with the signalling molecules such as receptors, non-receptor kinases, and Ras proteins. The mutations generally lead to constitutive signalling in the absence of a ligand and the signalling molecule does not shut off; it becomes uncoupled from normal growth control mechanisms.

Another method for oncogenic activation involves deregulated or inappropriate expression. This is generally seen with the nuclear proteins such as Myc. Since many of the nuclear proteins are induced by signals from extracellular sources, it would be reasonable to expect that overexpression of a nuclear oncogene might bypass the need for a signal in the first place. Deregulated expression can be achieved in a number of ways including gene amplifications and chromosomal translocations. Both gene amplification and chromosomal translocations involving proto-oncogenes have the net result of increasing the expression or deregulating the expression of a gene that is normally under tight controls.

Still another method for oncogenic activation of a proto-oncogene is by loss of a gene or loss of gene function. Proto-oncogenes that are activated in this manner are called suppressor genes or anti-oncogenes. Suppressor gene inactivation is generally seen as a result of chromosome deletions or mutations. Examples of suppressor genes are the retinoblastoma susceptibility gene, p53 and Wilms tumor gene.

COOPERATIVE TRANSFORMATION

It takes activation of more than one oncogene to convert a normal cell into a tumor cell.[10] At least two hits are required. This implies cooperativeness between oncogenes and is compatible with the multistage theory of carcinogenesis in which both initiating and promoting agents contribute to tumor formation. Cooperativeness between these agents is not random. For instance, as a rule, oncogenes which are activated by mutations of Ras and Src will cooperate with an oncogene activated by deregulated expression of Myc. Thus, Ras and Src do not cooperate but Ras and Myc or Src and Myc will. It is likely that cooperating oncogenes activate distinct or separate signal pathways, both of which must be activated to overcome normal cellular controls.

REGULATION OF GENE EXPRESSION

Several of the nuclear oncogenes can be classified as immediate early response genes in that transcription of these genes is rapidly turned on in response to a variety of signals. Until recently, the function of the nuclear oncogenes was not clear. It was known that they could bind to DNA but none had been shown to bind with any specificity. The c-Jun proto-oncogene was the first to be shown to contain sequence specific DNA binding ability and to act as a transcription factor. Although Jun was only isolated in 1987,[11] it has become one of the best characterized of the nuclear oncogene family. This was due to a number of important observations. The first was that the v-Jun oncoprotein shared homology with the yeast transcription factor GCN4.[5] The homology was limited to the carboxyl terminal third of each of the proteins that comprised the DNA binding domain of GCN4. The second observation was that the consensus target binding sequence of GCN4 - TGACTCA - is identical to the recognition sequence of the human transcription factor AP-1. This lead to the hypothesis that AP-1 and Jun were related. It was later shown that the c-Jun oncoprotein bound DNA with identical specificity to AP-1.[6] Evidence had been mounting that c-Fos oncoprotein also was associated with binding specifically to a TGACTCA sequence motif.[12] The Fos protein had been found associated with a cellular protein called P39. It was later shown that P39 and c-Jun were identical.[13] Thus, the products of two nuclear proto-oncogenes interact to form a transcription complex that is capable of regulating target gene expression. The nature of the interaction between Fos and Jun was found to be through a dimerization motif termed the leucine zipper.[14] The oncoproteins, *jun* and *fos*, belong to multigene families and all of the Fos family members can interact with all of the Jun family members.[15] In addition, all of the *jun* family members can dimerize with each other. Thus, the many different combinations of protein-protein interactions that occur, which allow regulation depending on the specific interaction, may regulate a number of shared targets - in addition to a number of unique targets.

Since the discovery of specific DNA binding with Jun and Fos, a number of other nuclear oncogenes have been shown to also have sequence specific DNA binding and transcriptional activation capabilities. These include c-Myc, c-Myb and c-Rel.

SUMMARY

In this short overview of oncogenes and cell growth, the protein products have been divided into two classes, proto-oncogenes and oncogenes. Proto-oncogenes can be activated by point mutations and deletions. Two classes exist: the dominant, which leads to cell growth and the suppressor, which by definition suppresses growth. The mechanism of action is multiplex - duplication of hormone action, resemblance to receptors, or kinases and DNA binding proteins.

It is clear that the regulation of cell growth and differentiation is very complex and that the products of proto-oncogenes play important roles in this regulation. Their functions appear to be at two levels. The first level is that of transduction of signals to the nucleus where the signals can be acted upon. The second is at the level of specific gene regulation, where incoming signals are turned into a response by the cell through activation of specific genetic programs. Nuclear proto-oncogene products play intimate roles in activation of these programs. The nature of the specific target genes regulated in response to these oncogene and proto-oncogene products however, remains a critical area of intensive research.

REFERENCES

1. R.F. Doolittle, M.W. Hunkapiller, L.E. Hood, S.G. Devare, K.C. Robbins, S.A. Aaronson, and H.N. Antoniades, Simian sarcoma virus onc-gene, v-sis, is derived from the gene (or genes) encoding a platelet-derived growth factor, Science. 221:275-77 (1983).
2. J. Downward, Y. Yarden, E. Mayes, G. Scrace, N. Totty, P. Stockwell, A. Ullrich, J. Schlessinger, and M.D. Waterfield, Close similarity of epidermal growth factor receptor and v-erbB oncogene protein sequences, Nature. 307:521-27 (1984).
3. C.J. Sherr, C.W. Rettenmier, R. Sacca, M.F. Roussel, A.T. Look, and E.R. Stanley, The c-fms proto-oncogene product is related to the receptor for the mononuclear phagocyte growth factor, CSF-1, Cell. 41:665-76 (1985).
4. K. Damm, C.C. Thompson, and R.M. Evans, Protein encoded by v-erbA functions as a thyroid-hormone receptor antagonist, Nature. 339:593-97 (1989).
5. P.K. Vogt,, T.J. Bos, and R.F. Doolittle, Homology between the DNA-binding domain of the GCN4 regulatory protein of yeast and the carboxyl-terminal region of a protein coded for by the oncogene jun, Proc Natl Acad Sci USA. 84:3316-19 (1987).
6. D. Bohmann, T.J. Bos, A. Admon, T. Nishimura, P.K. Vogt, and R. Tjian, Human proto-oncogene c-jun encodes a DNA binding protein with structural and functional properties of transcription factor AP-1, Science. 238:1386-92 (1987).
7. C.J. Marshall, Tumor suppressor genes, Cell. 64:313-26 (1991).
8. J.L. Bos, Ras oncogenes in human cancer: a review, Cancer Research. 49:4682-89 (1989).
9. H. Riedel, J. Schlessinger, and A. Ullrich, A chimeric ligand binding v-erbB/EGF receptor retains transforming potential, Science. 236:197-202 (1987).
10. T. Hunter, Cooperation between oncogenes, Cell. 64:249-70 (1991).
11. Y. Maki, T.J. Bos, C. Davis, M. Starbuck, and P.K. Vogt, Avian sarcoma virus 17 carries the jun oncogene, Proc Natl Acad Sci USA. 84:2848-52 (1987).
12. R.J. Distel, H.S. Ro, B.S. Rosen, D.L. Groves, and B.M. Spiegelman, Nucleoprotein complexes that regulate gene expression in adipocyte differentiation: direct participation of c-fos, Cell. 49:835-44 (1987).
13. F.J. Rauscher III, D.R. Cohen, T. Curran, T.J. Bos, P.K. Vogt, D. Bohmann, R. Tjian, and R.R. Franza Jr., Fos-associated protein p39 is the product of the jun proto-oncogene, Science. 240:1010-16 (1988).
14. W.H. Landschulz, P.F. Johnson, and S.L. McKnight, The leucine Zipper: A hypothetical structure common to a new class of DNA binding proteins, Science. 240:1759-64 (1988).
15. P.K. Vogt and T.J Bos, Oncogene and transcription factor. Adv Cancer Res. 55:1-35 (1990).

DISCUSSION

D. LeRoith: I haven't followed the literature and I'm not sure I understand. Are you saying that 27 base pairs from the tail into the V-jun interferes with it's translation?

T. Bos: In the transcription assays?

D. LeRoith: Yes.

T. Bos: You were shown that when the 27 amino acids are present transcriptional activation is decreased.

D. LeRoith: So it actually contained the V-jun?

T. Bos: Yes.

T. Lauterio: You showed reversion back to V-jun. How does that affect transformation?

T. Bos: Transformation is decreased when the 27 amino acids are present.

T. Lauterio: Does it behave more like C-jun in that instance?

T. Bos: Yes.

J. Nielsen: Do you know whether phosphorylation is involved?

T. Bos: Phosphorylation is involved, but exactly how it is involved I'm not sure. Along with the point mutations in the carboxyterminal region, one of these is serine/ phenylalamine mutation which is a GSK-3 kinase phosphorylation site. Actually, that particular serine residue has to be phosphorylated before 2-4 more serines and threonines can be phosphorylated so that apparently affects phosphorylation significantly. However, it doesn't seem to affect transformation.

INTERFERON - A CANDIDATE MEDIATOR OF CELL GROWTH

Bruce Tedeschi[1]

[1]Eastern Virginia Medical School
Department of Anatomy and Neurobiology
Norfolk, VA 22501

INTRODUCTION

Interferon (IFN) was originally discovered in 1958, when it was found that extracts of virally infected cells conferred anti-viral resistance in host cells.[1] Since the discovery of IFN, it has become clear that there are at least three antigenically defined families of IFNs (IFN-β, IFN-γ, and IFN-α) and that such IFNs have diverse, pleiotropic effects on IFN receptor-bearing host cells.[2-3] Some of these host cell effects include the modulation of cell growth and the induction of antigens of the Major Histocompatibility Complex (MHC). The ability of IFNs to stimulate the expression of MHC antigens suggests that they could be involved in the immunopathological responses of tissues to disease or injury. This may be the case for the destruction of islet β cells in the diabetic pancreas[4] or demyelination of CNS neurons in multiple sclerosis.[5] In this chapter, however, the ability of CNS cells to produce (and, or make biological responses to) IFN in the context of normal developmental processes and proliferation will be used as a model to illustrate the scope for IFN action. Studies of CNS injury and development at the molecular level might have implications for similar functions in the pancreas.[6]

IFN EXPRESSION AS A GENERAL CELLULAR RESPONSE TO GROWTH FACTOR STIMULATION

Can normal biological activities induce the expression of IFN from certain tissues? Current data suggest that the induction of IFN expression might be a specific response of some cells to growth factor stimulation. For example, in growth-quiescent 3T3 cells, the addition of platelet derived growth factor (PDGF), which elicits cell cycle-competence in quiescent G0 cells, initially stimulates the expression of several gene products including c-myc[7] and c-fos.[8] A somewhat delayed response of 3T3 cells to the addition of PDGF was the induction of IFN-β gene expression.[9] These investigators suggested that IFN-β might negatively feed back on the cell population to intrinsically down-regulate the proliferative response of the cells to the growth factor. Furthermore, they found that double-stranded RNA, which induces the expression of IFN-α/β stimulates the same set of early competence gene products in 3T3 cells as does PDGF. These data suggest a very close relationship between induction of IFN and growth factor stimulation.

This relationship between growth factors and IFN is not unique to PDGF, the 3T3 cell line, or *in vitro* studies. A pheochromocytoma tumor cell line (PC-12), popular for studies of neuronal differentiation since it responds to the presence of nerve growth factor (NGF) by mitotic arrest with subsequent differentiation into a neuronal phenotype,[10] expresses an IFN-β-like gene product following exposure to NGF.[11] These data suggest that the *in vitro* induction of IFN by growth factors may be a general phenomenon. These *in vitro* observations have been corroborated *in vivo*. Resnitzky et al[12] found that colony stimulating factor 1 induces the expression of IFN-β and that the secreted IFN is then associated with subsequent growth inhibition and hematopoietic cellular differentiation. These data lend credence to the hypothesis that IFN might function in many tissues or organs as an anti-growth factor playing a role in the regulation of normal cell growth.

EXPRESSION OF IFN BY CNS NEURAL CELLS

Early studies demonstrated the presence of IFN in cerebrospinal fluid (CSF) following viral infection of the CNS.[13-15] Since IFN normally cannot cross the blood-brain-barrier,[16,17] these experimental findings may reflect viral-induced changes in cerebrovascular permeability allowing IFN to enter the CNS parenchyma. Alternatively, the presence of IFN in CSF could be due to the secretion of IFN by CNS neural cells. We, therefore, sought to determine whether specific neural cells *in vitro* could be induced to express IFN in response to viral-like stimuli.[18] When purified cultures of mouse cortical astrocytes were incubated *in vitro* with double-stranded RNA, a stimulus known to induce IFN from non-neural cells,[2-3] titratable units of secreted IFN were observed. This IFN, secreted from astrocytes, was found to display physicochemical and immunological properties of the IFN-α/β class. When astrocytes were incubated with phytohemagglutinin or concanavalin A (stimuli known to induce IFN-γ from T lymphocytes), no titratable IFN was observed. The induction of IFN-α/β from astrocytes did not appear to be a non-specific, trivial response since no measurable IFN was inducible in cultured CNS cortical neurons. These data provided strong support that certain CNS neural cells have the capacity to produce IFN in response to viral-like stimuli.

We have obtained preliminary evidence that IFN is inducible by growth factors in neural cells.[19] When purified growth-quiescent cultures of mouse cerebral cortical astrocytes were stimulated to divide by epidermal growth factor (EGF), we observed the subsequent induction of IFN-α/β. Further, in immunohistochemical studies utilizing polyclonal IFN-α/β antisera, we have demonstrated IFN-α/β immunoreactivity in cryostat tissue sections of optic nerve.[19] In similar studies, Schmidt et al[20] have reported the *in vivo* expression of IFN-γ in optic nerve. This is an unusual finding since it was previously believed that IFN-γ was exclusively expressed by T cells. More definitive proof of *in vivo* IFN expression by CNS neural cells will probably require the cellular localization of IFN mRNA by in situ hybridization studies.

BIOLOGICAL RESPONSES OF CNS NEURAL CELLS TO IFN

Both CNS glial cells (astrocytes, oligodendrocytes, microglia) and neurons upregulate the expression of MHC antigens in response to IFN-α/β and/or IFN-γ.[11,21,22] Thus, it is clear that most CNS neural cell types probably bear receptors for one or all of the classes of IFN. Other responses of CNS neural cells to IFN are currently ill-defined. Since most IFN receptor-bearing cells respond to IFN by modulation of cell growth, it would perhaps not be surprising to find that the proliferation of some CNS neural cells can be regulated by IFN. Secreted factors (e.g. IFN), which control the proliferation of CNS cells, would play major roles in CNS development and responses to injury. For example, during optic nerve development, the differentiation of a bipotential progenitor cell into either a type-2 astrocyte or oligodendrocyte depends on the relative presence of two growth factors (PDGF and ciliary neurotrophic factor).[23] If PDGF only is present, the progenitor cell will divide a fixed number of times and apparently cease division autonomously and differentiate into an oligodendrocyte. The signals which are responsible for this autonomous growth inhibition following growth factor stimulation are not known, but IFNs (or other molecules with similar properties) could certainly account for this developmental phenomenon.

In the adult CNS, a consequence of injury is the proliferation of normally quiescent astrocytes and the appearance of larger, intermediate filament-packed glial cells. This inflammatory response has been called reactive gliosis and the resulting glial scar may play a role in the inability of damaged CNS axons to regenerate.[24] It has been shown that IFN-γ promotes both the proliferation of adult astrocytes *in vitro* and reactive gliosis *in vivo*.[25] Although these data suggest that IFN could contribute to reactive gliosis following injury, it is not clear whether IFN directly induces such changes or acts through its effects on the production of other cytokines. This is an important distinction since other cytokines (e.g. interleukin-1) are known to have growth-stimulatory effects on neural cells.[26] It is also not known whether, in certain cases, IFN-α/β can also be growth stimulatory for neural cells.

A final important biological response of CNS cells to IFN may be the facilitation of cell survival. It is known that primary cultures of sympathetic neurons are totally dependent on NGF in the growth medium for their survival. Martin et al[27] showed that death of cultured sympathetic neurons by NGF depletion appeared to be an apoptotic process since the death profile of the cell population could be partially inhibited by metabolic inhibitors. Another study demonstrated that IFN-γ, but not other cytokines, also promoted sympathetic neuronal survival *in vitro* when NGF was removed from the growth medium and that these sympathetic neurons displayed specific IFN-γ-binding receptors.[28] These results demonstrated that both NGF and IFN-γ can inhibit cell death (apoptosis) in sympathetic neurons, possibly by regulating utilization of metabolic substrates in neurons. A potential common pathway, regulated by both NGF and IFN-γ, is the activation of the enzyme oligo-2'5'-synthetase.[29] One function of oligo-2'5'-synthetase is to activate a latent cellular ribonuclease, RNase L.[3] Hence, NGF and IFN-γ might inhibit the expression of cell death RNA by operating on the oligo-2'5' -synthetase and RNase L pathway. Alternatively, both factors could be acting at a metabolic step removed from cell death RNA. Although these data suggest that IFN can regulate neuronal survival, it remains to be shown whether IFN plays such a role *in vivo*.

SUMMARY

The IFNs are a class of compounds comprising at least three different entities α, β, γ, with a clearly defined capacity to enhance expression of MHC antigens, as well as modulate growth in a variety of tissues. They are thus candidates for autoimmune cellular destruction **and** growth modulation.

IFN has now been shown to modulate important developmental and injury-related events in both the pancreas and CNS. Other cytokines may also be important players in these biological events and it remains to be elucidated how IFN and other cytokines exert their effects in these organs.

REFERENCES

1. A. Isaacs, J. Lindenmann, Virus interference: I - The interferon, Proc R Soc Lond [Biol]. 147:258-67 (1957).
2. S. Pestka, J.A. Langer, K.C. Zoon, C.E. Samuel, Interferons and their actions, Ann Rev. Biochem., Vol. 56, C.C. Richardson, P.D. Boyer, I.B. Dawid, and A. Meister, eds., (1987).
3. E. De Maeyer, J. De Maeyer-Guignard, "Interferons and Other Regulatory Cytokines," Wiley, New York (1988).
4. N. Sarvetnick, J. Shizuru, D. Liggitt, T. Stewart, Inflammatory destruction of pancreatic β cells in γ-interferon transgenic mice, *in:* "Cold Spring Harbor Sympositum," Quant. Biol. 54:837-842, 1989.
5. U. Traugott, E.L. Reinherz, C.S. Raine, Multiple sclerosis-distribution of T cell subsets within the active chronic lesions, Science. 219:308-10 (1983).
6. N.E. Sarvetnick, this volume.
7. K. Kelley, B.H. Cochran, C.D. Stiles, P. Leder, Cell-specific regulation of the c-myc gene by lymphocyte mitogens and platelet-derived growth factor, Cell. 35:603-10 (1983).
8. M.E. Greenberg, E.B. Ziff, Stimulation of 3T3 cells induces transcription of the c-fors proto-oncogene, Nature. 311:433-42 (1984).
9. J.N. Zullo, B.H. Cochran, A.S. Huang, C.D. Stiles, Platelet-derived growth factor and double-stranded ribonucleic acids stimulate expression of the same genes in 3T3 cells, Cell. 43:793-800 (1985).
10. L.A. Greene, A.S. Tischler, Establishment of a noradrenergic clonal line of rat adrenal pheochromocytoma cells which respond to nerve growth factor, Proc Natl Acad Sci USA. 73:2424-28 (1976).
11. F. Tirone, E.M. Shooter, Early gene regulation by nerve growth factor in PC12 cells: induction of an interferon-related gene, Proc Natl Acad Sci USA. 86:2088-92 (1989).
12. D. Resnitzky, A. Yarden, D. Zipori, A. Kimchi, Autocrine β–related interferon controls c-myc suppression and growth arrest during hematopoietic cell differentiation, Cell. 46:31-40 (1986).

13. L.B. Allen, K.W. Cochran, Target-organ treatment of neurotropic virus disease with interferon inducers, Infect Immun. 6:819-23 (1972).
14. F. Cathala, S.J. Baron, Interferon in rabbit brain, cerebrospinal fluid and serum following administration of polyinosinic-polycytidylic acid, Virology. 14:1355-58 (1970).
15. W.E. Stewart II, S.E. Sulkin, Interferon production in hamsters experimentally infected with rabies virus, Proc Soc Exp Biol Med. 23:650-53 (1966).
16. A. Billiau, Interferon therapy-pharmacokinetic and pharmacological aspects, Arch Virol. 67:121-33 (1981).
17. Y. Kono, M. Ho, The role of the reticuloendothelial system in interferon formation in the rabbit, Virology. 25:162-65 (1965).
18. B. Tedeschi, J.N. Barrett, R.W. Keane, Astrocytes produce interferon that enhances the expression of H-2 antigens on a subpopulation of brain cells, J Cell Biol. 102:2244-53 (1986).
19. B. Tedeschi, F.J. Liuzzi, C.W. Morgan, Expression of murine interferon in the central nervous system, Soc Neurosci Abstr. 17:754.
20. B. Schmidt, G. Stoll, K.V. Toyka, H.P. Hartung, Rat astrocytes express interferon-gamma immunoreactivity in normal optic nerve and after nerve transection, Brain Res. 515:347-50 (1990).
21. L.A. Lampson, C.A. Fisher, Weak HLA and β_2-microglobulin expression of neuronal cell lines can be modulated by interferon, Proc Natl Acad Sci USA. 81:6476-80 (1984).
22. G.H.W. Wong, P.F. Bartlett, I. Clark-Lewis, J.L. McKimm-Breschkin, J.W. Schrader, Interferon-gamma induces the expression of H-2 and Ia antigens on brain cells, J Neuroimmunol. 7:255-78 (1985).
23. L.E. Lillien, M.C. Raff, Analysis of the cell-cell interactions that control type-2 astrocyte development *in vitro*, Neuron. 5:111-19 (1990).
24. P.J. Reier and J.D. Houle, The glial scar: Its bearing on axonal elongation and transplantation approaches to CNS repair, *in:* "Functional Recovery in Neurological Diseases. Advances in Neurology", v. 47 S.G. Waxman (ed), Raven Press, New York, pp.87-138 (1988).
25. V.W. Yong, R. Moumdjian, F.P. Yong, T.C.G. Ruijs, M.S. Freedman, N. Cashman, J.P. Antel, Gamma-interferon promotes proliferation of adult human astrocytes *in vitro* and reactive gliosis in the adult mouse brain *in vivo*, Proc Natl Acad Sci USA. 88:7016-20 (1991).
26. D. Giulian, T.J. Baker, Characterization of ameboid microglia isolated from developing mammalian brain, J Cell Biol. 101:2411-15 (1985).
27. D.P. Martin, R.E. Schmidt, P.S. DiStefano, O.H. Lowry, J.G. Carter, Inhibitors of protein synthesis and RNA synthesis prevent neuronal death caused by nerve growth factor deprivation, J Cell Biol. 106:829-44 (1988).
28. J.Y. Chang, D.P. Martin, E.M. Johnson, Interferon suppresses neuronal cell death caused by nerve growth factor deprivation, J Neurochem. 55:436-45 (1990).
29. M. Saarma, U. Toots, E. Raukas, A. Zhelkovesky, A. Pivazian, T. Neuman, Nerve growth factor induces changes in (2'-5') oligo (A) synthetase and 2'-phosphodiesterase activities during differentiation of PC12 pheochromocytoma cells, Exp Cell Res. 166:229-36 (1986).

DISCUSSION

T. Lauterio: You indicated that neurons cannot be induced to produce interferon gamma or the MHC antigen.

B. Tedeschi: Yes, other investigators have claimed that neurons can produce a subset of MHC antigens, but we have not found that in our system.

T. Lauterio: Is it clear that there is no evidence from any investigators for interferon production by neurons?

B. Tedeschi: That's correct.

T. Lauterio: I suggest that, perhaps, you guys are looking in the wrong place for the neurons. The place I would suggest is an area implicated in the neuronal-glial interaction that would be the most likely to show interferon. So it seems to me, you would look at hypothalamic rather than cortical structures.

B. Tedeschi: Well, I don't know if the production of interferon by neurons is necessarily so important. I mean the neurons are intricately associated with the environment and they respond to their environment and they have receptors for response to that environment. Neurons are obviously closely associated with astrocytes and their supporting cells. The fact that these cells are capable of producing interferons and at least for what appears to be cell death and cell survival, neurons appear to have receptors to these molecules, I think that is the critical concept.

D. LeRoith: What you showed us early on - the neurons and the astrocytes - are these neonatal?

B. Tedeschi: That's right. The neurons have to be grown in embryonic form and we took them at E-15 and in mouse. The astrocytes can be taken at various points in time but definitely not after one day.

D. LeRoith: Have you tried culturing the adults?

B. Tedeschi: No. Some people have planned to culture adults but they don't do very well. What are the implications?

D. LeRoith: We have been culturing astrocytes, the adult astrocytes and looking at IGF effects on function. I was wondering what would happen to adult astrocytes in the sense that IGF tends to affect survival. But you haven't done that?

B. Tedeschi: Seeing whether the adult astrocytes will respond would be interesting. The astrocytes in culture, even for long periods of time, are capable of being induced to produce interferon, even cultured for periods of maybe 30 - 60 days.

D. LeRoith: Do you leave your embryonic or neonatal astrocytes in culture for a long time?

B. Tedeschi: They can be cultured for a long time. That's right.

D. LeRoith: Then they are not really embryonic any more. They have probably changed?

B. Tedeschi: Yes, if you think that the developmental program is ongoing *in vitro*.

C. Newgard: I may have missed this, but how do you get rid of the oligos from the astrocyte in culture?

B. Tedeschi: That is a very good question. I am basically using the following technique: Plate the cells in a T-75 flask. After about 8 or 9 days, you will find a lawn of platter cells that are your astrocytes. And on top of that lawn are these - we call them "fried eggs" that adhere loosely. A lot of these procedures are based on relative adherence of different cell types to different supporting media. When you look at some other cells, you'll see differences in adherence to tissue culture plastic versus collagen substrates. Well, as it turns out the oligodendrites are that population of cells that are loosely adhering to the top of this lawn. After about 8 or 9 days, what you do then, is close your flask tight, shake it overnight on a shaker. The next day, pipette off that population and selectively plate on tissue culture plastic. Then replate the growing population on your collagen polylysine substrate and greater than 95% of those cells are GC positive. These are oligodendrocytes.

SECTION TWO

MODELS FOR THE STUDY
OF CELL REGENERATION

ISLET β-CELL REGENERATION AND *REG* GENES

Michiaki Unno, M.D.[1] Takako Itoh,[2] Takuo Watanabe, M.D., Ph.D.[1]
Hikari Miyashita, M.D.[1] Shigeki Moriizumi,M.D.[1] Hiroshi Teraoka,[2]
Hideto Yonekura, Ph.D[1] and Hiroshi Okamoto, M.D., Ph.D.[1,3]

[1]Tohoku University School of Medicine
 Department of Biochemistry
 Sendai 980, Miyagi, Japan

[2]Shionogi Research Laboratories
 Shionogi & Co. Ltd.
 Osaka 553, Japan

[3]Tohoku University of Medicine
 Department of Biochemistry
 2-1 Seiryo-machi, Aoba-ku
 Sendai 980, Miyagi, Japan

INTRODUCTION

We have proposed a unifying model for the action of alloxan and streptozotocin on pancreatic β-cells.[1-5] Central to the model are breaks in the nuclear DNA of β-cells resulting from either an accumulation of oxygen radicals or alkylation of DNA. These breaks induce DNA repair involving the activation of poly(ADP-ribose) synthetase, which uses cellular NAD as a substrate; as a result, intra-cellular levels of NAD fall dramatically. The fall in cellular NAD inhibits the cellular activities including insulin synthesis, thus the β-cell ultimately dies.

Interest in the model for the mechanism of action of alloxan and streptozotocin has been heightened by the possible extension to the effects of viruses and inflammation, especially immune-mediated variants.[3-5] It is possible to assume that although insulin-dependent (Type I) diabetes can be caused by many different agents such as immunologic abnormalities, inflammatory tissue damage, and b-cytotoxic chemical substances such as alloxan and streptozotocin, the final pathway for the toxic agents is the same. This pathway involves DNA damage, poly (ADP-ribose) synthetase activation, NAD depletion, and inhibition of cellular activities. Therefore, insulin-dependent (Type I) diabetes is theoretically preventable through suppressing immune reactions, scavenging free radicals, and inhibiting poly(ADP-ribose) synthetase activity by enzyme inhibitors such as nicotinamide and 3-aminobenzamide.[3-5] An alternative consideration is the degree of ß-cell regeneration associated with β-cell destruction. If mechanisms regulating the regenerative response could be established, then this would be a feasible alternative.

β-CELL REGENERATION IN PARTIALLY DEPANCREATIZED ANIMALS

Current techniques for experimental diabetes in animals are mostly based on use of b-cytotoxins such as alloxan and streptozotocin. An alternative approach, following von Mering and Minkowski,[6] is to perform a partial pancreatectomy. Furthermore, from a practical point of view, strategies for influencing the replication of islet β-cells and the growth of the β-cell mass, in order to ameliorate not only insulin-dependent (Type I) diabetes but also non-insulin-dependent (Type II) diabetes, may be important. This type is not the result of an ongoing destruction of islet β-cells, but may reflect the inability of the β-cells to meet an increased peripheral demand for insulin.

In 1984, we demonstrated that poly (ADP-ribose) synthetase inhibitors induce regeneration of pancreatic β-cells, thereby preventing surgical diabetes.[7] Male Wistar rats were 90% depancreatized, and beginning 7 days before the partial pancreatectomy and continuing postoperatively, nicotinamide (0.5 g/kg body weight) or 3-aminobenzamide (0.05 g/kg body weight) was injected intraperitoneally every day. As shown in Figure 1, in 90% depancreatized rats, active DNA replication was observed in the islet β-cells of the remaining pancreas for 15 days. The regenerative process in the β-cells, however, did not continue further and the β-cells degenerated. In rats that were 90% depancreatized and treated with a poly(ADP-ribose) synthetase inhibitor, the replicative DNA synthesis increased and the β-cells continued to regenerate. In rats receiving poly (ADP-ribose) synthetase inhibitors, the urinary glucose excretion level decreased markedly.[7] Plasma glucose levels in rats receiving poly (ADP-ribose) synthetase inhibitors were also significantly lower than those in control 90% depancreatized rats. The islets in the remaining pancreases of rats which had received the poly(ADP-ribose) synthetase inhibitor for 3 months were very much larger than those in the control, and almost the entire area of the enlarged islet was densely stained for insulin. These results indicated that poly(ADP-ribose) synthetase inhibitors induced pancreatic β-cell regeneration, thereby ameliorating diabetes caused by a partial pancreatectomy.[2-5,7]

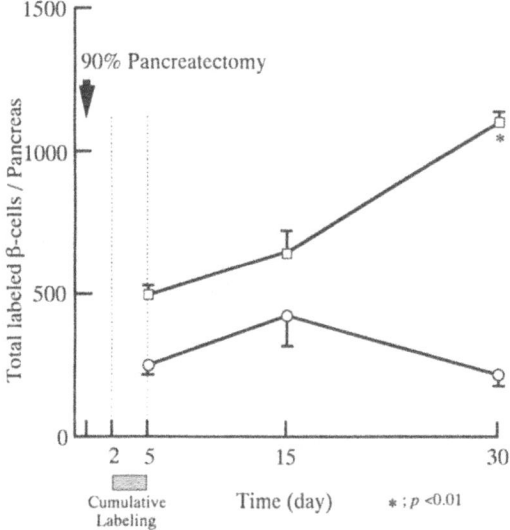

Figure 1. Cumulative labeling autoradiography for the quantitative estimation of β-cell proliferation and β-cell loss.[8,9] Ninety percent depancreatized rats receiving 3-aminobenzamide (□) or saline (○) given intraperitoneally at a dose of 0.5 μCi/g ³H-thymidine every 8 hours from 24 to 120 hours. The results are described as mean ± S.D.

REGENERATING GENE, *REG*

In 1988, we isolated regenerating islets from 90% depancreatized and poly(ADP-ribose) synthetase inhibitor-treated rats and constructed a cDNA library. In screening the regenerating islet-derived cDNA library, we came across a novel gene expressed in regenerating islets.[10] The cDNA had one large open reading frame which encoded a 165-amino acid protein (Figure 2). The deduced protein has a putative signal sequence. We proposed naming the novel gene *reg*, i.e., regenerating gene, with the implication that the gene may be involved in islet regeneration. *Reg* was expressed in regenerating islets, but not in normal islets.[10,11] Itoh et al[12] have constructed a yeast expression vector, in which a cDNA sequence encoding rat *reg* proteinexpressed in regenerating islets, but not in normal islets.[10,11] Itoh et al[12] have constructed a yeast expression vector, in which a cDNA sequence encoding rat *reg* protein was placed under the control of the PHO5 promoter. The construct was used to transform a yeast *Saccharomyces cerevisiae* strain AH22. The yeast produced a rat *reg* protein of 16 kDa without the signal peptide and secreted it into a culture medium. We purified the 16 kDa protein and prepared an antibody against it. Terazono et al[13] examined the localization of the *reg* protein in normal and regenerating rat islets using immunocytochemical techniques. Normal islets were densely stained for insulin. However, in a thin serial section, normal islets were not stained for the *reg* protein. Two weeks after the 90% pancreatectomy and nicotinamide treatment, regenerating islets were stained for *reg* protein. The immunostaining for the *reg* protein exhibited a distribution pattern almost identical to that of insulin-positive cells in a thin serial section of the regenerating islets. It should be noted here that some exocrine cells in regenerating and normal pancreases were also stained for the *reg* protein:[13] this staining in exocrine cells will be discussed later. One year after the 90% pancreatectomy and nicotinamide treatment, the islet cells were scarcely stained for *reg* protein, but the islets showed an immunoreactivity for insulin comparable to that of normal islets. In the double immunocytochemical staining, the *reg* protein was stained with large gold particles and insulin was stained with small gold particles. Both insulin and *reg* protein were electron microscopically found to be co-localized in the secretory granules of the regenerating β-cells.[13] These results suggested that the *reg* protein was synthesized in and secreted from regenerating β-cells, and that the expression of *reg* was closely associated with ß-cell regeneration.

```
                      Signal sequence

RAT          1  MTRNKYFILLSCLMVLSPSQGQEAEED-------LPSARI
MOUSE  I     1  MARNAYFILLSCLIVLSPSQGQEAEED-------LPSARI
MOUSE  II    1  MAQNNVYLILFLCLMFLSYSQGQVAEEDFPLAEKDLPSAKI
HUMAN        1  MAQTSSYFMLISCLMFLSQSQGQEAQTE-------LPQARI


TCPEGSNAYSSYCYYFMEDHLSWAEADLFCQNMNSGYLVSVLSQAEGNFLASLIK
SCPEGSNAYSSYCYYFTEDRLTWADADLFCQNMNSGYLVSVLSQAEGNFVASLIK
NCPEGANAYGSYCYYLIEDRLTWGEADLFCQNMNAGHLVSILSQAESNFVASLVK
SCPEGTNAYRSYCYYFNEDRETWVDADLYCQNMNSGNLVSVLTQAEGAFVASLIK


ESGTTAANVWIGLHDPKNNRRWHWSSGSLFLYKSWDTGYPNNSNRGYCVSVTSNS
ESGTTDANVWTGLHDPKRNRRWHWSSGSLFLYKSWATGSPNSSNRGYCVSLTSNT
ESGTTASNVWTGLHDPKSNRRWHWSSGSLFLFKSWATGAPSTANRGYCVSLTSNT
ESGTDDFNVWIGLHDPKKNRRWHWSSGSLVSYKSWGIGAPSSVNPGYCVSLTSST


GYKKWRDNSCDAQLSFVCKFKA      165
GYQKWKDDNCDAQYSFVCKFKG      165
AYKKWKDENCEAQYSFVCKFRA      173
GFQKWKDVPCEDKFSFVCKFKN      166
```

Figure 2. Alignment of the amino acid sequences of rat, mouse(I and II) and human *reg* proteins deduced from the cDNA sequences. Amino acids are given in the single-letter code.

ISOLATION OF TWO KINDS OF *REG* GENES FROM THE MOUSE GENOME

More recently, we have isolated two kinds of *reg* homologues from mouse pancreatic transcripts.[14] We designated the two *reg* homologues *reg* I and *reg* II, respectively. *Reg* I had one large open reading frame which encoded a 165-amino acid protein having a 21-amino acid signal sequence. *Reg* II encoded a 173-amino acid protein that had a 7-amino acid sequence in the amino-terminal region, as shown in Figure 2. At the amino terminus of the *reg* II protein, there was a signal sequence which was one amino acid longer than that of the *reg* I. In the optimally matched alignment, there was 76% homology in nucleotide and 75% homology in amino acid sequences between the *reg* I and *reg* II. We isolated the mouse *reg* I and II genes from the genomic DNA library and determined the complete nucleotide sequences and analyzed the mouse genomic DNA by Southern blot hybridization using the intron sequences as probes. The results showed that each *reg* gene was composed of six exons spanning about 3 kbp and present as a single copy in a haploid set of the mouse genome.[15]

We have already reported that aurothioglucose induced islet hyperplasia in NON mice.[10,11] The standard NON mouse spontaneously displayed impaired glucose tolerance. Aurothioglucose administration to NON mice caused islet hyperplasia, thereby ameliorating the glucose intolerance. Immunocytochemical examination showed that the hyperplastic islets consisted predominantly of β-cells. We examined the expression of the mouse *reg* I and II genes in hyperplastic islets, normal islets and normal whole pancreases by Northern blot hybridization using the synthetic oligonucleotides specific to the *reg* I or II cDNA as probes. Both *reg* I and II mRNAs were detected in the hyperplastic islet and normal pancreas, but not in the normal islet. The amounts of *reg* I mRNA in the hyperplastic islet and in the normal pancreas were 5 times higher than that of *reg* II mRNA.

We have already isolated a human *reg* homologue encoding a 166-amino acid protein from a human pancreas-derived cDNA library.[10] Figure 2 shows a comparison of the amino acid sequences among the rat and human *reg* proteins and the two mouse *reg* proteins. The rat and human proteins lacked the 7-amino acid sequence that was present in the mouse *reg* II protein, and therefore they were similar to the mouse *reg* I protein. Watanabe et al[16] isolated the human genomic *reg* and determined the complete nucleotide sequence: the gene spanned about 3 kbp and consisted of six exons separated by five introns. In the Southern blot analysis of human genomic DNAs under conditions of low stringency, we observed some additional bands, hybridizing to the *reg* cDNA probe, that were not predictable from the restriction map of the gene. Therefore, it is possible that rat and human genomes contain the *reg* II gene or a *reg*-related sequence.

REG PROTEIN, PANCREATIC STONE PROTEIN (PSP) AND PANCREATIC THREAD PROTEIN (PTP)

Recently, two proteins named pancreatic stone protein (PSP) and pancreatic thread protein (PTP) were isolated from human pancreatic juice and pancreases and sequenced.[17-19] Since the primary amino acid sequence of PSP and PTP was identical with that of the protein encoded in the human *reg* gene, we have concluded that the *reg* protein, PSP and PTP, are the same protein that comes from the human *reg* gene and that PSP and PTP are the processed products of the *reg* protein.[16]

We examined the localization of the human *reg* protein or PSP in a normal human pancreas using the antibody against a human recombinant *reg* protein.[12] The human exocrine pancreas was densely stained for the *reg* protein, but the normal human islet was not stained by the antibody. In chronic pancreatitis, the localization of *reg* protein, when it occurred, was extremely weak in the exocrine cells, as already reported by Lechene de la Porte et al[20] who examined the localization using the antibody against PSP. It has been suggested that PSP prevents the formation of pancreatic stones,[21] and that PTP is a filamentous protein.[19] Hypothetically, therefore, when the expression of the *reg* gene is depressed, regeneration of endocrine β-cells may not proceed, and the decreased synthesis of PSP/PTP may lead to pancreatic stone formation and pancreatic fibrosis. This speculation seems to be of interest in understanding the pathogenesis of malnutrition-related diabetes mellitus,[22] because pancreatic stone formation and pancreatic fibrosis are associated with this form of diabetes,[23-25] and because the endocrine and exocrine components of the pancreas have been suggested to function together in morphogenesis and cell function.[26,27]

SUMMARY

In this paper, we show that the *reg* gene is expressed in experimentally induced regenerating or hyperplastic islets. We have previously reported that ectopic expression of the *reg* gene occurs in some human colonic and rectal tumors, suggesting that enhanced *reg* expression may be related to the proliferative state of tumor cells.[16] *Reg* protein has also been shown to have significant sequence homology with plant and animal lectins,[28] a class of compounds that has been shown to be a growth promoter. At present, any direct relationship between *reg* protein and β-cell replication remains to be established. However, since the *reg* protein is a secretory protein and *reg* can be expressed at an early stage of pancreatic cell differentiation, the *reg* protein may act on the stem cells of β-cells in an autocrine or paracrine manner. In normal mature exocrine cells, the *reg* gene is expressed and the gene product may be necessary to maintain adequate exocrine pancreatic function. The physiological reasons for the maintenance of two functional *reg* genes encoding proteins of slightly different sequence in mice are still unclear. The cloning of additional rat and human non-allelic *reg* genes could provide additional clues.

REFERENCES

1. H. Okamoto, Regulation of proinsulin synthesis on pancreatic islets and a new aspect to insulin-dependent diabetes, Mol Cell Biochem. 37:43-61 (1981).
2. H. Okamoto, Molecular basis of experimental diabetes: degeneration, oncogenesis and regeneration of pancreatic β-cell of islets of Langerhans, BioEssays. 2:15-21 (1985).
3. H. Okamoto, *Rig* and *reg* novel genes activated in insulinomas and in regenerating islets, *in:* "Diabetes 1988 - Proceedings of the 13th Congress of the International Diabetes Federation, Sydney, 20-25 November 1988", R.G. Larkins, P.Z. Zimmet, and D.J. Chishlm, eds., Excerpta Medica, Amsterdam (1989).
4. H. Okamoto, The molecular basis of experimental diabetes, *in:* "Molecular Biology of the Islets of Langerhans", H. Okamoto, ed., Cambridge University Press, Cambridge, (1990).
5. H. Okamoto, H. Yamamoto, S. Takasawa, C. Inoue, K. Terazono, K. Shiga, and M. Kitagawa, Molecular mechanism of degeneration, oncogenesis and regeneration of pancreatic β-cell of islets of Langerhans, *in:* "Frontiers in Diabetes Research: Lessons from Animal Diabetes II", E. Shafrir and A.E. Renold, eds., John Libbey & Company Ltd., London (1988).
6. J. von Mering, and O. Minkowski, Diabetes mellitus nach Pankreasexstripation, Arch Exp Pathol Pharmakol. 26:371-87 (1890).
7. Y. Yonemura, T. Takashima, K. Miwa, I. Miyazaki, H. Yamamoto, and H. Okamoto, Amelioration of diabetes mellitus in partially depancreatized rats by poly (ADP-ribose) synthetase inhibitors: evidence of islets β-cell regeneration, Diabetes. 33:401-04 (1984).
8. Y. Matsuda, Regeneration of β cells in partially depancreatized rats poly (ADP-ribose) synthetase inhibitor, Suizo (J Jpn Panc Soc.) 2:450-59 (1987).
9. Y. Yonemura, T. Takashima, T. Hashimoto, I. Miyazaki, H. Yamamoto, and H. Okamoto, β-cell replication in regenerating islets of 90% depancreatized poly (ADP-ribose) synthetase inhibitor-treated rats, Tonyobyo (J Jpn Diabetes Soc.) 28:363 (1985).
10. K. Terazono, H. Yamamoto, S. Takasawa, K. Shiga, Y. Yonemura, Y. Tochino, and H. Okamoto, A novel gene activated in regenerating islets, J Biol Chem. 263:2111-14 (1988).
11. K. Terazono, T. Watanabe, and Y. Yonemura, A novel gene, *reg*, expressed in regenerating islets, *in:* "Molecular Biology of the Islets of Langerhans", H. Okamoto, ed., Cambridge University Press, Cambridge (1990).
12. T. Itoh, H. Tsuzuki, T. Katoh, H. Teraoka, K. Matsumoto, N. Yoshida, K. Terazono, T. Watanabe, H. Yonekura, H. Yamamoto, and H. Okamoto, Isolation and characterization of human *reg* protein produced in *Saccharomyces cervisiae*, FEBS Lett. 272:85-88 (1990).
13. K. Terazono, Y. Uchiyama, M. Ide, T. Watanabe, H. Yonekura, H. Yamamoto, and H. Okamoto, Expresion of *reg* protein in rat regenerating islets and its co-localization with insulin in the ß-cell secretory granules, Diabetologia. 33:250-52 (1990).
14. M. Unno, T. Itoh, T. Watanabe, S. Moriizumi, H. Miyashita, K. Nata, T. Anzai, H. Yonekura, H. Teraoka, and H. Okamoto, The structure and expression of two mouse reg genes (*reg* I and *reg* II), Seikagaku. 63:1012 (1991) (Abstract in Japanese).
15. M. Unno, T. Itoh, T. Watanabe, H. Teraoka, H. Yonekura, and H. Okamoto, (1991) in preparation.
16. T. Watanabe, H. Yonekura, K. Terazono, H. Yamamoto, and H. Okamoto, Complete nucleotide sequence of human *reg* gene and its expression in normal and tumoral tissues, J Biol Chem. 265:7432-39 (1990).

17. A. De Caro, J.J. Bonicel, P. Rouimi, J.D. De Caro, H. Sarles, and M. Rovery, Complete amino acid sequence of an immunoreactive form of human pancreatic stone protein isolated from pancreatic juice, Eur J Biochem. 168:201-07 (1987).
18. A. De Caro, Z. Adrich, B. Fournet, C. Capon, J.J. Bonicel, J.D. De Caro, and M. Rovery, N-terminal sequence extension in the glycosylated forms of human pancreatic stone protein; the 5-oxoproline N-terminal chain is O-glycosylated on the 5th amino acid residue, Biochim Biophys Acta. 994:281-84 (1989).
19. J. Gross, R.I. Carlson, A.W. Brauer, M.N. Margolies, A.L. Warshaw, and J.R. Wands, Isolation, characterization, and distribution of an unusual pancreatic human secretory protein, J Clin Invest. 76:2115-26 (1985).
20. P. Lechene de la Porte, A. De Caro, H. Lafont, and H. Sarles, Immunocytochemical localization of pancreatic stone protein in the human digestive tract, Pancreas. 1:301-08 (1986).
21. L. Multigner, A. De Caro, Lombardo, D., Campese, D. and H. Sarles, Pancreatic stone protein, a phosphoprotein which inhibits calcium carbonate precipitation from human pancreatic juice, Biochem Biophys Res Commun. 110:69-74 (1983).
22. WHO Study Group, Diabetes Mellitus, World Health Organization Technical Report Series 727, Geneva, WHO (1985).
23. P.H. Bennett, Epidemology of diabetes mellitus, in: "Diabetes Mellitus-Theory and Practice, Fourth Edition," H. Rifkin and D. Porte Jr., eds., Elsevier, New York (1990).
24. S.S. Fajans, Classification and diagnosis of diabetes, in: "Diabetes Mellitus-Theory and Practice, Fourth Edition", H. Rifkin and D. Porte Jr., eds., Elsevier, New York (1990).
25. G. Montalto, L. Multigner, H. Sarles, and A. De Caro, Organic matrix of pancreatic stones associated with nutritional pancreatitis, Pancreas. 3:263-68 (1988).
26. R.N. Melmed, Intermediate cells of the pancreas, Gastroenterology. 76:196-201 (1979).
27. W.J. Rutter, R.L. Pictet, J.D. Harding, J.M. Chirgwin, R.J. MacDonald, and A.E. Przybyla, An analysis of pancreatic development: role of mesenchymal factor and other extracellular factors, in: "Molecular Control of Proliferation and Differentiation", J. Papaconstantinou and W.J. Rutter, eds., Academic Press, New York (1978).
28. L.A. Lasky, M.S. Singer, T.A. Yednock, D. Dowbenko, C. Fennie, H. Rodriguez, T. Nguyen, S. Stachel, and S.D. Rosen, Cloning of a lymphocyte homing receptor reveals a lectin domain, Cell. 56:1045-55 (1989).

DISCUSSION

A. Vinik	Hiroshi, as usual your report was magnificent and clearly communicated. I want to ask one little question. This model of yours was so interesting in terms of treatment with nicotinamide and aurothioglucose. If you followed the animals longer, because now, in terms of your theory you should have a lot of DNA that is fractured with the chemical insult, do they go on to develop tumors because of the abnormal DNA?
H. Okamoto:	I do not understand your question.
A. Vinik:	I mean, with long term treatment with nicotinamide and aurothioglucose, in your model do you see tumor formation? I am not questioning how it occurrs, necesarily. But if it occurs through a process that involves the abnormal or fragmented DNA which is then expressed in a form that manifests a tumor down the road rather than simply a hyperplastic islet which represents the adult type of islet.
H. Okamoto:	When we inject streptozotocin and nicotinamide into the rats we can easily induce insulinomas in rats. But in this case (nicotinamide and aurothioglucose) only one or two of the insulinomas are apparent.
C. Newgard:	I was just wondering if, in your immunocytochemistry is it at all possible that the Reg signal that you see in islets is produced in the exocrine tissue and is somehow transported to the islets and is decorating the surface of the cell. Would the conditions under which you did the immunocytochemistry allow you to see proteins decorating the surface of the cell?
H. Okamoto:	What do you mean by, "the proteins decorating?"
C. Newgard:	I mean, is it possible that the Reg that you seem to see in the autoradiography, is not within the cells but in adjacent tissues?
A. Vinik:	What he means is, when you see Reg expression it maybe in acinar tissue, not islets. That is to say, Reg is being synthesized in the exocrine cells and being moved into the islet and that is the reason it appears to be in the islet.
H. Okamoto:	No, in fact our data would argue against that.
A. Vinik:	So that would suggest that the protein is getting to the islet cell.
C. Newgard:	That's what I think, is the issue at hand.
H. Okamoto:	You may be correct, but we've isolated islets without acinar cells, and we detected Reg suggesting that it does derive from the islet.
C. Newgard:	You mean, amylase or elastase or any of these sorts of serine proteases?

C. Newgard:	I would argue that it is very, very difficult to isolate islets without contaminating endocrine tissue.
H. Okamoto:	We have separated islets from acinar cells and found reg within the islets.
C. Newgard:	Well, I'm going to show you a slide in which we used your model. What we see in some experiments is a halo of Reg expression surrounding the islet and it appears to be in the exocrine tissue immediately surrounding the islet. So this could also indicate (assuming there is the same degree of exocrine contamination in the two islet preparations) that Reg is induced in exocrine tissue immediately surrounding the islet. This could explain your results.
A. Vinik:	Are you going to show us the data using immunochemistry to prove that the protein actually appears within the islet.
H. Okamoto:	No, we have not been able to do that.
S. Bonner-Weir:	We've done immuncytochemistry and we don't see it in the regenerating islets.
A. Vinik:	Derek, you had a question.
D. LeRoith:	My question relates to the two genes, encoding Reg-1 and Reg-2. On one, Reg-1, you have a TATA box, and on the other you did not find a TATA box?
H. Okamoto:	No, we have now completed the sequence of Reg 2 and it does contain a TATA box.
J. Nielsen:	I would also add that we got antibody from Dr. Okomoto and tried it on the growth hormone-stimulated islet and didn't see any break in those islets. So I would ask a question related to stem cells. Do you think your regenerating islets come from ducts or do they come from the existing islets?
H. Okamoto:	Normal ducts contain Reg message.
J. Nielsen:	Did you look at embryonic development of the pancreas?
H. Okamoto:	We are studying the growth development of the pancreas.
R. Rafaeloff:	Since we know from other models that 90% pancreatectomy also leads to the same effect of spontaneous regeneration and expression of Reg, what exactly is nicotinamide doing or is it the same effect that spontaneous regeneration would do in this model?
H. Okamoto:	Please repeat the question.
A. Vinik:	She wants to know that if you see spontaneous regeneration, as Susan Bonner-Weir shows, with a 90% pancreatectomy, is nicotinamide doing anything over and above the pancreatectomy? More than the pancreatectomy alone.
S. Bonner-Weir:	Arthur, that will probably come out when I give my talk.
L. Rosenberg:	Is the Reg gene expression in your model an epi-phenomenon, or is it really responsible for the regeneration? And if you think it is responsible for the regeneration have you tried to culture islets in tissue culture and stimulate regeneration with Reg protein.

H. Okamoto:	Do you mean, does Reg protein stimulate growth of islets *in vitro*? We have tried to apply Reg protein to freshly isolated islets, but presently we have no evidence that it stimulates the growth of islets.
A. Vinik:	I think that we will have to accept that the involvement of Reg is, at best, indirect; there is no direct evidence that Reg is expressed in regenerating islets and there is direct evidence, as far as we know, at this point in time, that the administration of Reg protein to an animal made diabetic can actually reverse the diabetes.
H. Okamoto:	We did try to put some Reg protein into cultures with islet cells and measured for deoxyuridine incorporation and it didn't seem to have much of an effect, although it was very preliminary.
R. Rafaeloff:	When the Reg gene or pancreatic stone protein is expressed, do you think that this gene is differently regulated or has different regulatory mechanisms? Because if the gene is not expressed and you don't have the pancreatic stone protein it means that the animal will develop pancreatitis.
H. Okamoto:	We do think Reg gene is involved in regeneration. We cannot discuss a role related to pancreatic stone protein.

FACTORS REGULATING ISLET REGENERATION
IN THE POST-INSULINOMA NEDH RAT

Ling Chen, M.D.[1] Michael C. Appel, Ph.D.[2] Tausif Alam, Ph.D.[1]
Chisato Miyaura, Ph.D.[1] Andrea Sestak, B.S.[1] John O'Neil, B.S.[2]
Roger H. Unger, M.D.[1] and Christopher B. Newgard, Ph.D.[1,3]

[1]Center for Diabetes Research, Gifford Laboratories
Departments of Biochemistry and Internal Medicine
University of Texas Southwestern Medical Center
Dallas, TX 75235

[2]University of Massachusetts Medical Center
Department of Anatomy
Worcester, MA 01605

[3]Center for Diabetes Research, Gifford Laboratories
University of Texas Southwestern Medical Center
5323 Harry Hines Blvd.
Dallas, TX 75235

INTRODUCTION

Increases in islet β-cell mass can be induced in a variety of experimental models, and can also occur in the face of metabolic stress, such as obesity, or in certain genetic backgrounds such as the ob/ob mouse. The factors responsible for compensatory proliferation of islet β-cells are not understood, but as this volume attests, investigation in the area is intensifying. Our own work has heretofore utilized the insulinoma-bearing New England Deaconess Hospital (NEDH) rat[1] as a model for studying islet regeneration.[2,3] Implantation of a solid insulinoma tumor into NEDH rats causes dramatic suppression of the mass and function of their islet β-cells; this suppression is reversed rapidly by surgical removal of the tumor.[2,3] We have used this model system to address two specific issues. First, we have investigated the regulation and site of expression of the *reg* gene, which was cloned by Okamoto and coworkers in 1988[4] by virtue of its preferential expression in a cDNA library prepared from isolated islets taken from 90% pancreatectomized, nicotinamide-injected rats, an alternate model of β-cell regeneration.[4,5] The primary sequence of *reg* was subsequently shown to be identical to that of the pancreatic stone protein (PSP),[6-8] an exocrine gene product whose only known function is to inhibit $CaCO_3$ crystal growth, thus helping to prevent chronic calcifying pancreatitis.[9-13] Second, we have begun to develop differential screening strategies designed at identifying other genes that might be involved in the expansion of β-cell mass. These initiatives are reviewed herein, and new data on the site of expression of *reg*/PSP is also provided.

The Tumor-Bearing NEDH Rat

The major advantages of the tumor-bearing NEDH rat model are 1) Islet regeneration is rapid, and can thus be studied without the necessity for prolonged animal manipulation, and 2) A selective regeneration of β-cells is achieved without physical manipulation of the pancreas, making it less likely that changes observed are artifacts of surgery. Figure 1 provides a schematic summary of the experimental model employed in our studies as well as the metabolic and morphological consequences of tumor implantation and removal. Experiments are begun by transplantation of a small insulinoma tumor into the scapular region of the host animals, and as the tumor grows over the ensuing 7-10 weeks, the animals become increasingly hypoglycemic and hyperinsulinemic in response to the insulin produced by the tumor. Meanwhile, the animal's own islet β-cells become increasingly atrophic and reduce their insulin production. In our studies, blood glucose is monitored daily, and the animals are kept at 20-30 mg/dl for 1 week prior to tumor removal in order to attain full suppression of β-cell mass and function. After this period of severe hypoglycemia, tissue and blood samples are taken at intervals following surgical removal of the tumor. The removal of the tumor results in transient hypoinsulinemia and hyperglycemia (persisting for the first 24-48 hours), followed by a return of these metabolic parameters to normal, as islet insulin production resumes.[2,3]

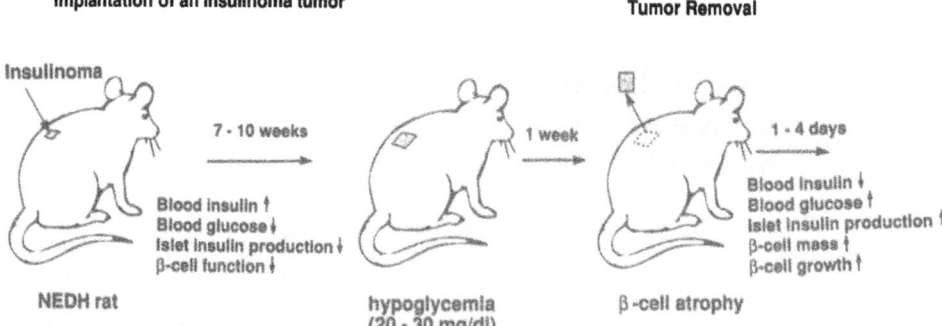

Implantation of an insulinoma tumor

Tumor Removal

Insulinoma

7 - 10 weeks

Blood insulin ↑
Blood glucose ↓
Islet insulin production ↓
β-cell function ↓

NEDH rat

1 week

hypoglycemia
(20 - 30 mg/dl)

1 - 4 days

Blood insulin ↓
Blood glucose ↑
Islet insulin production ↑
β-cell mass ↑
β-cell growth ↑

β-cell atrophy

Figure 1. The post-insulinoma NEDH rat as an experimental model of induced β-cell growth. Experiments are begun by implantation of a small transplantable insulinoma tumor in the scapular region. As the tumor grows over the ensuing 7-10 weeks, the animal becomes increasingly hyperinsulinemic and hypoglycemic, and decreases in endogenous islet insulin production and β-cell function are noticed. The animals are maintained in a severely hypoglycemic state (20-30 mg/dl) for one week prior to tumor resection, leading to marked islet atrophy due to a reduction in β-cell mass. Upon tumor removal, the islet β-cell mass returns to normal over a period of 4-5 days, in part because of a sharp increase in β-cell mitotic activity.

Appel and coworkers have made a careful study of the effect of tumor implantation and removal on islet β-cell morphology, mass and replication.[2,3] β-cells comprise 75-80% of the volume of the intact islet in normal rats. Implantation of an insulinoma tumor by the protocol described above results in a reduction of β-cell mass to where it comprises only 5-30% of the volume of the islet (i.e., non β-cells are predominant in the suppressed islet). As shown in Table 1, islet β-cell replication, measured *in vivo* by administration of ^{3}H thymidine and quantitation of grain-labeled nuclei in β-cells, is severely depressed in tumor-bearing animals. This value is even lower than the value for normal β-cells, which are known to have a low rate of turnover. Upon removal of the tumor, thymidine incorporation into β-cells increases dramatically, with a sharp peak of activity observed three days after tumor resection. β-cell volume, in contrast, increases in roughly linear fashion in response to tumor removal, and normal β-cell mass is reached 4-5 days after surgery. Our interpretation of this data is that the regeneration of islet β-cell mass in the post-insulinoma NEDH rat is a process comprised jointly of an increase in the volume of pre-existing cells, due in part to the increase in insulin biosynthesis and the regranulation of cells, and an increase in mitotic activity. Based on the data presented in Table 1, we conclude that volume changes make the predominant contribution to increased β-cell mass at days 1 and 2 after tumor resection, and that β-cell replication plays a larger role in the period from 2-4 days after surgery. It is appreciated that the differential screening strategies summarized below directed at isolating factors that orchestrate the increase in β-cell mitotic activity may also lead to cloning of genes that respond to, or are involved in, changes in cell volume.

Table 1. Animals received ^{3}H-thymidine intraperitoneally and were sacrificed 4 hours later. Pancreata were excised and processed for paraffin embedding. Prepared sections were immunostained with anti-glucagon, somatostatin, and pancreatic peptide antibodies collectively. Following autoradiography, the number of grain labeled nuclei seen in unstained (β) cells were counted. Results are expressed per 100 cells counted.

Days after Tumor Resection	Number of animals	% β-cells labeled
0	5	$0.06 \pm .001$
1	5	$0.09 \pm .003$
2	4	$0.83 \pm .018$
3	5	$6.14 \pm .820$
4	4	$0.80 \pm .086$
5	4	$0.76 \pm .008$
NEDH Controls	4	$0.73 \pm .010$

Recent experiments suggest that the effect of tumor implantation may be mediated by the attainment of low glucose concentrations. Maintenance of normal blood glucose concentrations in the face of an implanted insulinoma tumor prevents islet atrophy, and infusion of glucose into tumor-bearing animals with suppressed islets restores β-cell mass and function to normal.[2,14] Chronic insulin infusion for up to 12 days, a procedure that maintains blood glucose at around 50 mg/dl in our hands, fails to reduce islet β-cell mass significantly,[15,16] showing that insulin *per se* has no effect on islet atrophy, at least over the time period studied, and that only the more severe hypoglycemia (20-30 mg/dl) attained after 7-10 weeks of tumor implantation causes suppression. It remains possible, however, that other peptides or metabolites secreted by the tumor could also play a role.

Regulation of Expression of *reg*/PSP in the Tumor-Bearing NEDH Rat Model

Despite the demonstration of exact sequence identity of *reg* and pancreatic stone protein (PSP), a previously characterized pancreatic exocrine gene thought to comprise as much as 10% of the protein in exocrine secretions, we felt that characterization of *reg*/PSP expression in our model would be of interest for several reasons. First, Okamoto and colleagues had clearly demonstrated increased expression of the *reg* gene in isolated islet preparations from two models of islet regeneration, 90% pancreatectomized, nicotinamide injected rats, and in rats treated with aurothioglucose.[4] Second, *reg*/PSP has significant sequence homology with plant and mammalian lectins,[17,18] some of which have been ascribed a growth promoting role. Third, it seems possible that the dispersion of islets throughout the pancreas reflects a requirement for a factor or substance produced in exocrine cells that somehow nurtures or affects the function of the endocrine component, and that *reg*/PSP might be an example of such a factor.

A portion of our data on the effect of tumor implantation and removal on *reg*/PSP expression, summarized in complete detail elsewhere,[3] is presented in Table 2. We found that tumor implantation induced a dramatic suppression in *reg*/PSP mRNA levels in whole pancreas explants relative to pancreas samples taken from normal (non-tumor bearing) or sham surgery control NEDH rats (sham surgery refers to creation and religation of a surgical incision in the scapular region of a size similar to that needed for tumor removal, under pentobarbital anesthesia, 24 hours prior to pancreas removal). Tumor resection resulted in a

Table 2. *Reg*/PSP and Elastase mRNA Levels in Tumor-Bearing NEDH Rats Before and 24 Hours After Removal of the Insulinoma.

A.	*reg*/PSP mRNA		Elastase I mRNA	
	Tumor In	Tumor Out	Tumor In	Tumor Out
Pair 1	1	7.5	1	0.5
Pair 2	1	3.2	1	0.9
Pair 3	1	8.7	1	0.7
Pair 4	1	6.6	1	0.6

B.	Normal	Sham-Surgery	Normal	Sham-Surgery
Pair 5	7.2	7.6	0.9	1.1
Pair 6	9.0	10.0	1.3	1.3

Panel A. Age-matched pairs of animals were studied either in the presence of an insulinoma tumor (Tumor In) or 24 hours after surgical removal (Tumor Out). *reg*/PSP and elastase mRNA levels were determined by densitometric scanning of northern blots (see reference 3 for primary data) and are normalized to the signal obtained with an 18S ribosomal RNA probe. For each pair, the *reg*/PSP or elastase I mRNA level in the "tumor in" rat was normalized to 1 and the "tumor out" value is expressed as the multiple. Panel B. Pancreata were excised from age-matched pairs of normal animals that were either untreated or studied 24 hours after "sham" surgery. All values in panel B are normalized to the *reg*/PSP or elastase measurement for the tumor-bearing animal in pair 1 of panel A.

transient restoration of *reg*/PSP expression within 24 hours (Table 1) that persisted through 48 hours but then began to decline, reaching its nadir 3 days after tumor resection and then returning towards normal levels again 7 days after tumor resection (the later time points are not shown in Table 1 but are presented in reference 3). Interestingly, chronic insulin infusion for a period of 4 days, a maneuver that strongly suppresses pancreatic insulin mRNA levels but has little effect on islet β-cell mass,[15,16] also had no effect on *reg*/PSP mRNA levels compared to saline infused controls.[3]

Table I also shows that in contrast to *reg*/PSP, elastase I mRNA levels are unaffected in tumor-bearing animals relative to normals, and are reduced rather than elevated in response to tumor removal. We have since expanded the study to include a number of other exocrine genes and find that kallikrein, trypsin I, amylase, elastase II, and chymotrypsin expression are either unaffected or only slightly changed in response to tumor implantation and removal, suggesting that the large changes seen in *reg*/PSP mRNA levels do not reflect a global increase in exocrine gene expression.[19]

Site of expression of *reg*/PSP

Prior to the first report of sequence identity of *reg* and PSP, Ling Chen and co-workers had observed preferential expression of *reg*/PSP mRNA in pancreatic acinar cells rather than in islets, using the technique of *in situ* hybridization.[20] Later, we used this technology to show that tumor resection causes a dramatic increase in the *reg* mRNA signal that appeared to be mostly confined to exocrine tissue, although a low level of expression in islets could not be excluded. When the sequence identity of *reg* and PSP was brought to light, these data were easily understood, since the French group that originally discovered PSP had used immunological techniques to establish its expression in exocrine tissues and secretions.[11-12] Despite the mounting evidence for exocrine expression of the gene, Okamoto and colleagues, while conceding expression in acinar cells, recently reported that the *reg* gene product is also detected in islets during regeneration induced by pancreatectomy and nicotinamide injection.[21] Below we present further evidence for preferential, if not exclusive, expression of *reg*/PSP in the exocrine rather than the endocrine pancreas.

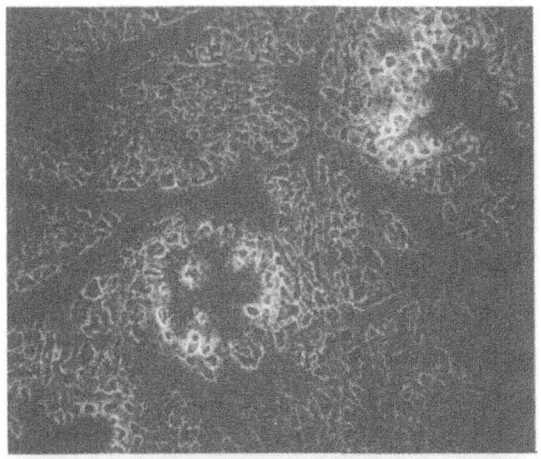

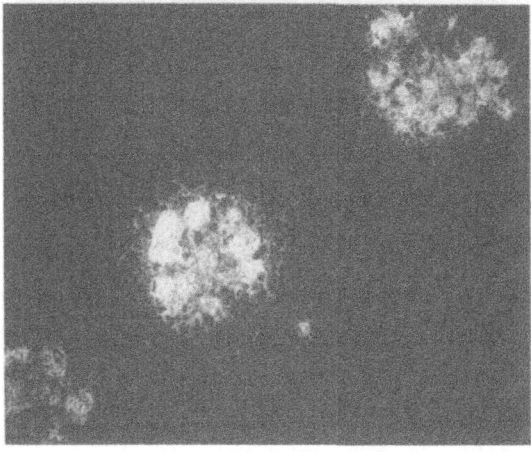

Figure 2. *In Situ* hybridization for *reg*/PSP in pancreas sections. Top: Dark-field photomicrograph of adjacent sections of a pancreatic remnant from a rat subjected to 90% partial pancreatectomy and nicotinamide injection, hybridized *in situ* with *reg*/PSP (top) and insulin antisense oligonucleotide probes (bottom). Note that the islets are devoid of *reg*/PSP signal, which is confined to exocrine cells. Although the section shows a perinsular distribution of signal, in other pancreata a more diffuse distribution of signal throughout acinar tissue was noted. The bar below the figure represents 500 μM.

Figure 2 demonstrates the tissue distribution of *reg*/PSP mRNA in sections of pancreas obtained from rats 12 weeks after 90% pancreatectomy and nicotinamide treatment to reproduce precisely the experimental protocol employed by Terazono et al.[4] Clearly the mRNA is confined to the exocrine tissue; the islets contain no more than the background level of signal. In some pancreata the signal was largely peri-insular in location (as shown in the example of Figure 2), while in others it was distributed throughout the pancreas. A similar pattern was observed in 90% pancreatectomized animals injected with saline instead of nicotinamide (data not shown). Islets were markedly enlarged in size and were irregular (see Figure 2), often having a stellate configuration relative to islets in pancreatic sections of normal animals. This is presumably the consequence of intrusion of regenerating endocrine tissue into the exocrine pancreas.

We also examined the site of expression of *reg*/PSP in human pancreas obtained at autopsy, using an antibody raised against purified human PSP.[11-12] As shown in Figure 3, immunofluorescence was confined to exocrine tissue, with no staining of endocrine cells.

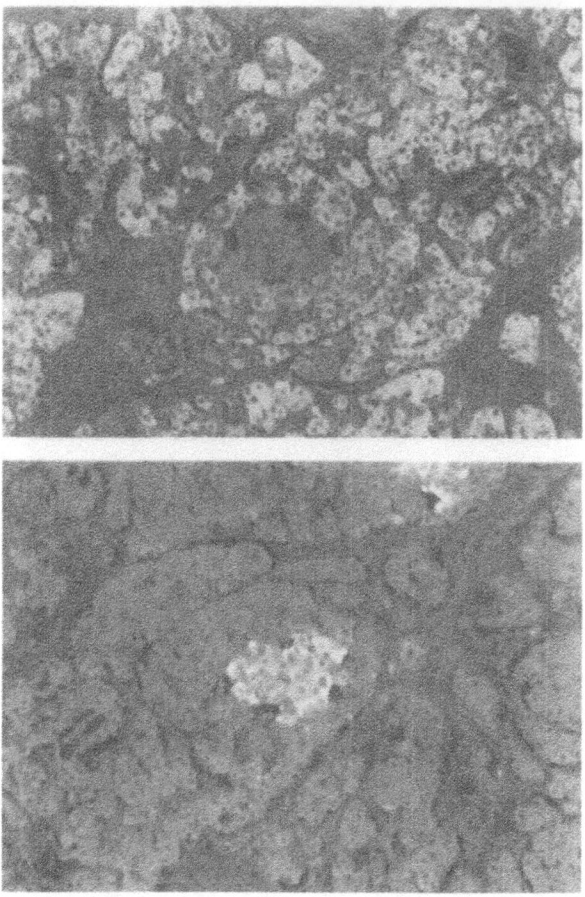

Figure 3. Immunocytochemistry of reg/PSP protein in human pancreas. A pair of consecutive serial sections of a normal human pancreas obtained at autopsy and stained by immunofluorescence with anti-reg/PSP antibodies (top) and anti-insulin antibodies (bottom). No evidence of reg/PSP immunofluorescence is noted within the islet, the signal being confined to exocrine tissue.

A final line of evidence for exclusive expression of reg/PSP in the exocrine pancreas is provided in Figure 4. The availability of cells derived from both insulinoma and pancreatic exocrine tumors allowed us to evaluate reg/PSP expression in both cell types. There was no detectable reg/PSP mRNA in the insulinoma cells, whereas significant quantities were present in the exocrine cell line. Figure 4 also shows substantial expression of reg/PSP in islets isolated by collagenase digestion and Ficoll gradient centrifugation. Note, however, that amylase mRNA was also clearly detectable in the sample, indicating significant contamination of the isolates with exocrine tissue.

In sum, these as well as previous data provide strong evidence that expression of the reg/PSP gene is confined to the exocrine pancreas and does not occur in endocrine pancreas, even during islet regeneration. A probable explanation for the initial confusion as to the site of reg/PSP expression may be found in Figure 2, which reveals intermingling of exocrine and endocrine tissue in the regenerating islets of 90% depancreatized rats. Cross-sections of such stellate islets through their peripheries would show exocrine cells completely surrounded by projections of regenerating endocrine cells and would explain the report of positive immunostaining for reg/PSP "within" islets.[21] It might also explain why there was significant exocrine contamination of the isolated islets used for the regenerating islet cDNA library of Terazono et al.[3,20]

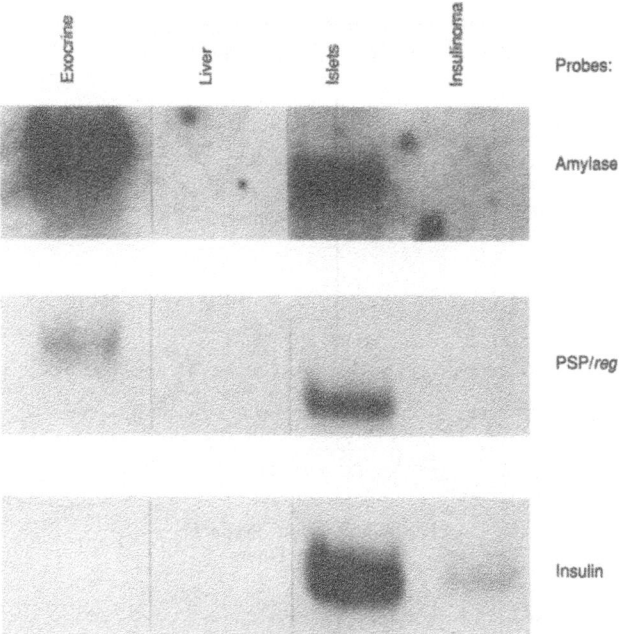

Figure 4. Blot hybridization analysis of steady state levels of *reg*/PSP, insulin, and amylase mRNas in various cell types. RNA was prepared and resolved as previously described.[3] Five mg of poly A+ RNA prepared from liver, isolated islets of Langerhans, or a solid insulinoma tumor, and 1 mg of poly A+ RNA prepared from the exocrine cell line AR42J ("exocrine") were loaded per lane, and the blot was hybridized sequentially with the indicated antisense probes.

Does *reg*/PSP Have a Role in Islet Regeneration?

Induced expression of *reg*/PSP has been reported in 3 unrelated experimental models of islet regeneration: 90% pancreatectomy in rats,[4] aurothioglucose treatment in mice,[4] and after removal of subcutaneously implanted insulinoma from NEDH rats.[3] Despite the fact that its expression generally parallels or precedes periods of islet mitotic activity in these models, other aspects of *reg*/PSP expression are difficult to reconcile with a β-cell cytotrophic role for this peptide, most notably its high level of expression in normal or sham-operated animals and the fact that PSP comprises as much as 10% of the protein in exocrine juice. During this symposium, mention was made of experiments in which the effect of the *reg*/PSP protein on primary islet cell proliferation was examined with no obvious effects. Despite the lack of direct evidence that *reg*/PSP directly influences β-cell growth, the concept that the exocrine pancreas, through specific trophic factors, provides a uniquely congenial environment for islets is an attractive one. The reports of a lack of direct effect of *reg*/PSP on isolated islets, when reported in full detail, will likely cause many to reject this protein as a participant in the process of β-cell regeneration. While this may ultimately prove to be the correct view, it remains possible that *reg*/PSP can affect islet β-cell growth in combination with other factors.

Molecular Approaches to Isolating Factors Regulating Islet Regneration in the Post-Insulinoma NEDH Rat

We have begun to employ techniques of molecular biology to clone cDNAs corresponding to mRNAs that are preferentially expressed during islet regeneration in the post-insulinoma rat model. Our initial approach involved differential screening of a cDNA library prepared from whole pancreas isolated 1 or 2 days following tumor resection. The strategy employed for differential screening of such libraries is shown in Figure 5 and can be

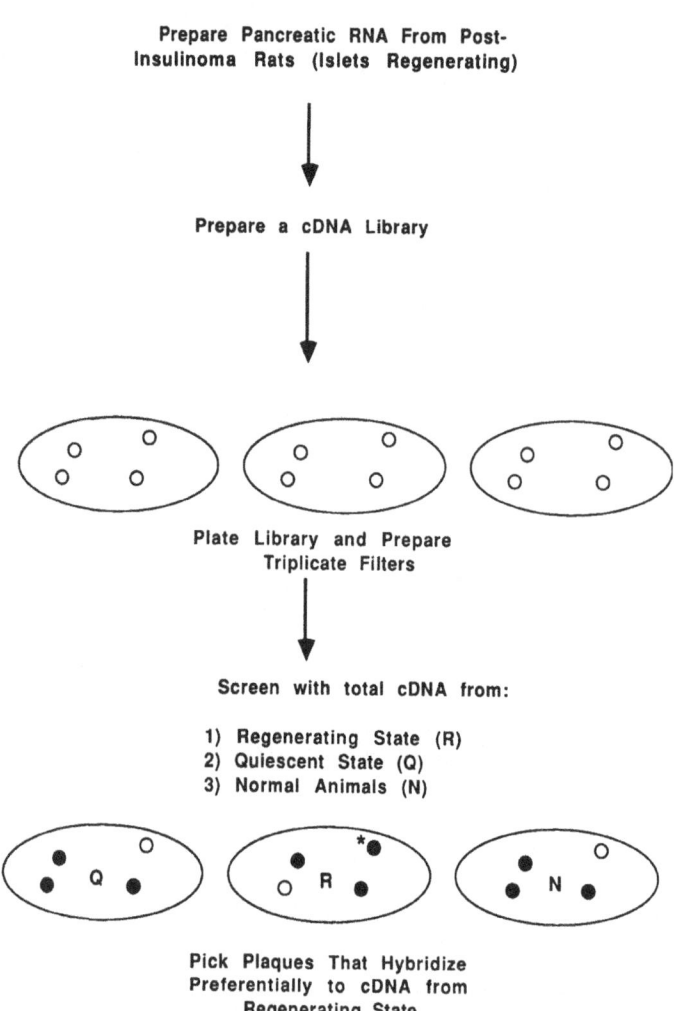

Figure 5. Strategy for Preparation and Screening of a cDNA Library Prepared From Whole Pancreas Containing Regenerating Islets.

summarized as follows: 1) Poly A$^+$ RNA was isolated from total pancreas samples harvested from normal animals (N), tumor-bearing animals (T), and post-insulinoma animals with regenerating islets (R). 2) A λgt10 cDNA library, consisting of 3.3 x 10^6 independent recombinants was prepared from the pancreatic RNA isolated from post-insulinoma rats (R) and screened with radiolabeled N, T, and R total cDNA samples. Clones hybridizing preferentially with R cDNA relative to N and T were isolated and subjected to sequence analysis.

Screening of approximately 15,000 recombinant plaques by this method resulted in the isolation of 2 distinct clones (several copies of each were found). One of the clones was identical to *reg*/PSP, underscoring the strongly induced expression of this gene following tumor resection. The second class of clones (termed 48-3) isolated by our screening strategy encodes a serine protease-like gene product. A time course study of 48-3 mRNA levels revealed that both normal and tumor-bearing animals expressed very low levels of this mRNA, but that tumor resection caused a 3.2-fold and a 4-fold increase at 1 and 2 days, respectively, after tumor removal; thereafter levels of this transcript declined gradually between days 3 through 7, finally reaching the low normal level. This pattern of expression is distinct from *reg*/PSP, which is expressed at a relatively high level in normal animals. We conclude that the pattern of expression of clone 48-3 is unique compared with other exocrine gene products included in the study and might be consistent with a role for this gene in islet regeneration.

The foregoing strategy is not optimal for the isolation of autocrine factors, i.e., factors produced by the islets themselves, because of the overwhelming predominance of exocrine RNA in the sample used to prepare the library. In order to circumvent this problem, we have recently prepared a cDNA library from islets isolated 72 hours after tumor resection (the period of maximum β-cell mitotic activity). A limiting factor for this approach is the difficulty encountered in obtaining islets. We have overcome this problem by developing a modification of the rapid amplification of cDNA ends (RACE) PCR technique of Frohman et al.[22] Total RNA was prepared from approximately 5,000 islets, and reverse transcribed with an oligo-dT primer which had an Eco RI site built in at its 5' end. After removal of the primer by filtration, a poly A tail was added to the first strand cDNA, and this material was subjected to PCR with the same oligo-dT Eco RI primer as used for first strand synthesis.

ACKNOWLEDGEMENTS

We thank Dr. Jean-Charles Dagorn (INSERM, Marseille) for providing the anti-PSP antibody, Dr. Ray MacDonald for the amylase cDNA, and Dr. Lindsey Inman for human pancreas samples. The work was supported by Juvenile Diabetes Foundation International (Grant 190727), NIH Grant DK-02700-30, and Veterans Administration Institutional Research Grant 549-8000.

REFERENCES

1. W.L. Chick, S. Warren, R.N. Chute, A.A. Like, V. Lauris, and K.C. Kitchen, A transplantable insulinoma in the rat, Proc Natl Acad Sci USA. 74:628-32 (1977).
2. F.J. Bedoya, F.M. Matschinsky, T. Shimizu, J.J. O'Neil, and M.C, Appel, Differential regulation of glucokinase activity in pancreatic islets and liver of the rat, J Biol Chem. 261:10760-64 (1986).
3. C. Miyaura, L. Chen, M. Appel, T. Alam, L. Inman, S.D. Hughes, J.L. Milburn, R.H. Unger, and C.B. Newgard, Expression of reg/PSP, a pancreatic exocrine gene: relationship to changes in islet β-cell mass, Mol Endocrinol. 5:226-34 (1991).
4. K. Terazono, H. Yamamoto, S. Takasawa, K. Shiga, Y. Yonemura, Y. Tochino, and H. Okamoto, A novel gene activated in regenerating islets, J Biol Chem. 263:2111-14 (1988).
5. H. Okamoto, Molecular basis of experimental diabetes: degeneration, oncogenesis, and regeneration of pancreatic b-cells of islets of langerhans, Bioessays. 2:15-21 (1985).
6. T.A. Stewart, The Human reg Gene Encodes Pancreatic Stone Protein, Biochem J. 260:622-23 (1989).
7. S. Rouquier, D. Giorgi, J. Iovanna, and J-C. Dagorn, Sequence similarity between the reg transcript and pancreatic stone protein mRNA, Biochem J. 264:621-24 (1989).
8. T. Watanabe, H. Yonekura, K. Terazono, H. Yamamoto, and H, Okamoto, Complete nucleotide sequence of human reg gene and its expression in normal and tumoral tissues: the reg protein, pancreatic stone protein, and pancreatic thread protein are one and the same product of the gene, J Biol Chem. 265:7432-39 (1990).
9. G. Montalto, J. Bonicel, L. Multigner, M. Rovery, H. Sarles, and A. DeCaro, Partial amino acid sequence of human pancreatic stone protein, a novel pancreatic secretory protein, Biochem J. 238:227-32 (1986).
10. A. DeCaro, L. Multigner, H. Lafont, D. Lombardo, and H. Sarles, The molecular characteristics of a human pancreatic acidic phosphoprotein that inhibits calcium carbonate crystal growth, Biochem J. 222:669-77 (1984).
11. P. Lechene de la Porte, A. DeCaro, M. Amouric, and H. Sarles, Localisation immunocytochemique del la proteine majoritaire des calculs pancreatiques humains, La Nouv Presse Med. 10:3851 (1981).
12. D. Giorgi, J-P Bernard, A. DeCaro, L. Multigner, R. Lapointe, H. Sarles, and J.C. Dagorn, Pancreatic stone protein. I. Evidence that it is encoded by a pancreatic ribonucleic acid, Gastroenterology. 89:381-86 (1985).
13. D. Giorgi, J-P Bernard, S. Rouquier, J. Iovanna, H. Sarles, and J-C Dagorn, Secretory pancreatic stone protein messenger RNA: nucleotide sequence and expression in chronic calcifying pancreatitis, J Clin Invest. 84:100-06 (1989).
14. M.C. Appel, unpublished data
15. L. Chen, I. Komiya, L. Inman, J. O'Neill, M. Appel, T. Alam, and R.H. Unger, Effects of hypoglycemia and prolonged fasting on insulin and glucagon gene expression, J Clin Invest. 84:711-14 (1989).
16. L. Chen, T. Alam, J.H. Johnson, S. Hughes, C.B. Newgard, and R.H. Unger, Regulation of ß-cell glucose transporter expression, Proc Natl Acad Sci USA. 87:4088-92 (1990).
17. T.E. Peterson, The amino-terminal domain of thrombomodulin and pancreatic stone protein are homologous with lectins, FEBS Lett. 231:51-53 (1988).
18. L. Patthy, Homology of pancreatic stone protein with animal lectins, Biochem J. 253:309-11 (1988).
19. Miyaura, C., Sestak, A., Appel, M. C., O'Neil, J., and Newgard, C. B., manuscript in preparation.

20. C. B. Newgard, S. Hughes, L. Chen, H. Okamoto, and J.L. Milburn, The *reg* gene is preferentially expressed in the exocrine pancreas during islet regeneration (abstract), Diabetes. 38:49A (1989).
21. K. Terazono, Y. Uchiyama, M. Ide, T. Watanabe, H. Yonekura, H. Yamamoto, and H. Okamoto, Expression of *reg* protein in rat renerating islets and its co-localization in the beta cell secretory granules, Diabetologia. 33:250-25 (1990).
22. M.A. Frohman, M.K. Dush, and G.R. Martin, Rapid production of full-length cDNAs from rare transcripts: amplification using a single gene-specific oligonucleotide primer, Proc Natl Acad Sci USA. 85: 8998-9002 (1988).

DISCUSSION

D. LeRoith: Chris, we go back a long way so I want to be a little bit critical, if you'll excuse me for just a minute.

C. Newgard: I would hope so.

D. LeRoith: Could you tell us a little bit more about this hypertrophy/hyperplasia that Arthur was asking about. To be a little bit more critical - and as we saw from the slides - there seems to be an increase of volume, and you spoke about DNA synthesis, but what you are really measuring is thymidine incorporation.

C. Newgard: Yes, that's right.

D. LeRoith: So, what I want to know is this: in those earlier days when there was perhaps hypertrophy - not hyperplasia - did you look at thymidine incorporation not just by looking at uptake of thymidine incorporation into TCA precipitable protein, but rather by incorporation of thymidine into DNA.

C. Newgard: No, no. It is not *in vivo*. This is how it's done. In the animal following tumor removal, an injection is given some period before - it's in the paper - either 12 or 24 hours before, and then sections are made and the beta cells are identified by staining with antibodies against glucagon and somatostatin. So, in other words, cells that don't stain are designated as beta cells. Then microscopic evaluation of the sections for grains of thymidine incorporation is done. So, it's not *in vivo*.

D. LeRoith: You know better than I do that thymidine incorporation isn't always into the DNA of the nucleus. So the question is, did you actually show hyperplasia by cell counting..

C. Newgard: I'll tell you that what Mike Apple has done is look at these sections rather carefully. He promises me that he sees multiple mitotic figures in the regenerative state as compared to either the quiescent state or earlier in regeneration when the thymidine incorporation is clearly lower than at day 3. What that implies also is that the proliferation is either in part, or largely, or in fact, all coming from pre-existing beta cells. He has seen mitotic figures in his evaluation of the sections.

D. LeRoith: The reason that I'd like to establish the point is that you mentioned earlier that the IGF-1 and IGF-1 receptor genes expressed are in the regenerating beta-cell. In my kidney regeneration model with hypertrophy - there is no IGF-1 or IGF-1 receptor, but there was in the hyperplasia and I wondered whether, when you did those studies, you looked at the stages where there was more hyperplasia than hypertrophy?

C. Newgard: No, we haven't.

D. LeRoith:	You haven't specifically looked at those then?
C. Newgard:	While we looked at the time course of the thymidine incorporation, we did not specifically address the issue of hyperplasia versus hypertrophy.
D. LeRoith:	I think that earlier on you might have more hypertrophy, and hyperplasia occurs later.
C. Newgard:	I wouldn't argue with that, I think I agree with you completely. I'm not trying to sell you the notion that this is a complete hyperplasia model. No, not at all.
D. LeRoith:	My question was: when did you look at the IGF-1 and IGF-1 receptors?
C. Newgard:	We looked in the full time course.
D. LeRoith:	And there was none?
C. Newgard:	Yes, we had trouble detecting it. Like Jens, I have trouble seeing it very well at all, although Susan is clearly showing their presence in her model of regeneration.
S. Bonner-Weir:	But ours is in focal regions in the pancreas. Ours is not related to islets per se, but ductal and vascular endothelial tissue.
C. Newgard:	We were doing RNAse protection assays and are still having trouble picking it up in pancreas RNA.
S. Bonner-Weir:	Well, we did in situ hybridization and solution hybridization assays.
A. Vinik:	Susan, yours is in the focal regions of regeneration and Newgard is looking at adult cell regeneration, so yours may be coming from your type 1 ductal growth as opposed to adult endocrine tissue.
S. Bonner-Weir:	Our localization of the IGF-1, mainly in focal regions is the embryological recapitulation.
C. Newgard:	I think if we can be general, yours is selective recapitulation, ours is not.
S. Bonner-Weir:	No, we have both; we do have both.
C. Newgard:	At least, Mike Appel, the guy doing the morphology has argued that it is a pre-existing beta cell-pool.
A. Vinik:	In other words, the consensus would be that recapitulation of the fetal development process might be associated with IGF-1.
C. Newgard:	Yes, yes exactly.
H. Okamoto:	I would like for you and the people who are present here to tell me: is there anyone who has confirmed that amylase or so-called exocrine-specific enzymes are not expressed in islets?
C. Newgard:	You mean, amylase or elastase or any of these sorts of serine proteases?
H. Okamoto:	Yes, is it possible that chains of exocrine enzymes also express in islets in small amounts?

H. Okamoto:	Yes, is it possible that chains of exocrine enzymes also express in islets in small amounts?
C. Newgard:	Let me tell you a very interesting thing. Ray McDonald is a colleague at our place and he evaluates the elastase promoter. He has found 3 elements in the elastase promoter that appear to be important for pancreas specific expression. When he takes those promoters - the elements - and mixes them, let's say you have element A, B, and C regions of DNA. If he takes different regions of these and cuts some out - I can't remember exactly -but if he takes out the B element, suddenly in a transgenic model he's getting expression of elastase in the islet. So I think there is a possibility that exocrine substances are expressed in the islet tissue. In the normal animal, when examined with antibodies against various serine protease chains - elastase, amylase, and others - there is no evidence of any staining in islets, but there appears to be some of the information necessary to direct islet expression in the promoter region, for example, of the elastase gene, which under normal conditions would appear to be masked or blocked. What does this mean in terms of developmental expression and can it be the turn on of some genes during certain periods of development? - It's a possibility!
A. Vinik:	I want to go back to this question that was raised earlier. Is there any way we can identify whether only cells derived from ducts form Reg as opposed to existing beta-cells? Have you tried to address that before?
C. Newgard:	I have not, and really I can't take any credit for this model, nor do I care to take any flack about it. But no, I think - and this may be a weak argument - that there are mitotic figures in islets that appear in the course of the regeneration phase which seem to correlate the data for thymidine incorporation with the numbers of mitotic figures.
N. Sarvetnick:	Are they in islets or in duct cells?
C. Newgard:	No, these are beta cells within the islets.
S. Bonner-Weir:	Actually, I know Mike's data pretty well, too, and what you see when a tumor is present is that you'll have islets in a very degranulated form, and that the granules make up an appreciable amount of the volume of cells, and I think he also measured insulin content and insulin message. So he's getting not only endocrine cells hypertrophying or returning to normal size, but he has a very dramatic number of cells replicating - existing beta cells replicating.
C. Newgard:	I wouldn't argue with that.
A. Vinik:	You see, we've raised another whole issue and Lawrence will talk about it later. That is, when you see beta cells replicating they seem to go through a phase where these cells become larger and larger and then assume the adult configuration. One would like to see islet hyperplasis accounting for the physical changes in this model. Then the percentage of cells does change a lot in terms of the relationship of this new cell mass to the existing mass when volume of islets is taken into account.
S. Bonner-Weir:	Oh, absolutely. Whatever the stimulus, we have hypertrophy and hyperplasia.
A. Vinik:	Have you had the opportunity, to look at the proteins that are expressed in this suppressed stage and at the stage where regeneration is seen - as Gary Pittenger will show later this afternoon,?

C. Newgard: Yes, Mike Apple in collaboration with Franz Cochenski have shown expression of proteins in the regenerating islets. If we're talking about Reg, the answer is no. If we're talking about proteins in general, there has been some study of islet specific proteins done by Mike Apple. For example, it is claimed that glucokinase disappears in the suppressed islet and reappears after removal of the tumor. But we have not looked at Reg, nor have we had a chance to look at elastase-3 proteins.

A. Vinik: Looking at the gene itself, certainly in the 5prime-flanking regions, simple modifications markedly alter the ability to produce insulin, but there also seem to be domains, which when altered, change the status from cell to cell leading to tumor formation. Nora Sarvetnick has done this fascinating work looking at the histo-compatibility gene in the transgenic mice and also created a transgene containing interferon gamma, attached to the insulin promoter. The gene finds its way into the beta-cells, causes destruction followed or attended by regeneration. We may not have to look much further than the insulin gene itself.

REGENERATION OF PANCREATIC ENDOCRINE CELLS
IN INTERFERON-GAMMA TRANSGENIC MICE

Nora E. Sarvetnick, Ph.D.[1] Dangling Gu, M.D.[1]

[1]The Scripps Research Institute

Department of Neuropharmacology

La Jolla, CA

INTRODUCTION

There has been an enormous amount of research on the destruction of pancreatic islets, especially the β-cells, a condition which leads to insulin-dependent diabetes mellitus. On the contrary, not as much emphasis has been placed on the development and the maintenance of this endocrine tissue. In order to understand fully the pathogenesis of diabetes, it is equally important to gain insights into the growth and potential regenerative aspects of pancreatic islets. The mammalian pancreas first appears as dorsal and ventral buds from the embryonic gut.[1-3] The rudimentary pancreas grows rapidly, increasing its length, and extends to the surrounding tissue. The endocrine cells are first detected either in the wall of ducts or adjacent to the newly formed ducts. They form clusters as they grow in size and are segregated from the ducts as islets of Langerhans. Under normal conditions, the pancreatic islets and ducts remain relatively quiescent with minimal cell turnover throughout adult life. In streptozotocin-treated animals, and in type 1 diabetes no further growth apparently occurs. It should be noted, however, that several exceptions have been recently reported. For example, in the mouse there is a transient increase in islet β–cell number and islet size during pregnancy.[4,5] An increase in islet size and β-cell hyperplasia also occurs in mutant ob/ob mouse one month after birth and persists throughout life. These enlarged islets are only seen along the pancreatic ducts while those islets situated away from the ducts appear normal.[5,6] Another example of β cell growth in adults is the transgenic mouse carrying SV 40 large T antigen (Tag) linked to the insulin regulator gene. The mice which inherit the Tag transgene all show hyperplasia of the islets some of which transform to β-cell tumors.[5,7] Another illustration of pancreatic growth and regenerative capacity is found in rats after a 90% pancreatectomy. In this pancreatectomized model, the regeneration occurs by proliferation of duct cells and by increasing replication of existing differentiated cells.[8,9] Growth and differentiation of ductal cells in mature hamsters into islet cells without tumor formation is also possible by saran-wrapping of the pancreas or by the administraatioon of an extract of cytosol of wrapped pancreas.[10] We want to present, in the following sections, an islet regenerating model displayed by a transgenic mouse strain harboring the lymphokine interferon-γ (IFN-γ) gene linked to human insulin promotor. The ins-IFN-γ transgenic mice suffer from pancreatic inflammation and progressive loss of islets 6-8 weeks after birth.[11,12] Here we demonstrate that concurrent to the destructive process, the pancreatic islets undergo rapid regeneration by replication of duct cells and subsequent differentiation into endocrine cells.

PANCREAS MORPHOLOGY OF INS-IFN-GAMMA MICE

Histologic features of pancreas from IFN-γ transgenic mice are characterized by the presence of a variable number of inflammatory cells beginning from one month after birth.[11,12] The inflamed lesions become progressively more severe with age. By the time the animals reach five months of age or older, extensive obliteration and destruction of islet and acinar structures are observed in addition to the massive infiltration of inflammatory cells. Meanwhile, as islets are much less frequently seen, the pancreatic ducts become more prominent and interstitial fibrosis becomes more obvious. In the very old mice, one year or over, the adipocytes begin to accumulate within the pancreatic tissue and in the area surrounding the organ near the major blood vessels. The most notable morphological feature of pancreas from a three-six months old transgenic mouse, especially in the central region where the organ receives its blood supply, is the extensive array of pancreatic ducts which dominate the whole microscopic field (Figure 1). The duct wall, which normally consists of a single-layer of epithelial cells, now appears lobulated or decorated with buds of variable cell mass that occur at different loci along its length. In some instances, the lobes or buds are seen to protrude into the lumen. Discrete clusters of cell aggregates that resemble normal islet morphology are seen in the vicinity of ducts, more so in the older animals, three-six months of age. Electron microscopic observations of pancreatic ducts reveal normal morphology of epithelial cells which border the lumen. The epithelial cells are joined at tight junctions and project numerous microvilli into the lumen. The ducts are limited by a basal lamina on the basal side. Endocrine cells, identified by the content of dense granules in their cytoplasm, are present along the duct especially where the lobes or buds are located. (Data not shown) All three major cell types (alpha α, beta β and delta δ) are present based on the morphology of hormone-containing granules. Interestingly, the endocrine cells often contain more than one type of dense granules in the same cell.

Identification of Different Phenotypes By An Immunolabeling Technique

The α, β, and δ, cell types of islets are identified by an immuno-peroxidase method using specific antibodies against each corresponding hormone - glucagon, insulin, and somatostatin -produced in each cell type. The results of these experiments, in agreement with the electron microscopic observations, show that all three cell types are present in the duct wall and in the islet-like cell mass (Figures 2, 3, 4).

Identification of Proliferation Cells

The replicating cells are labeled by the incorporation of thymidine analog, bromodeoxy

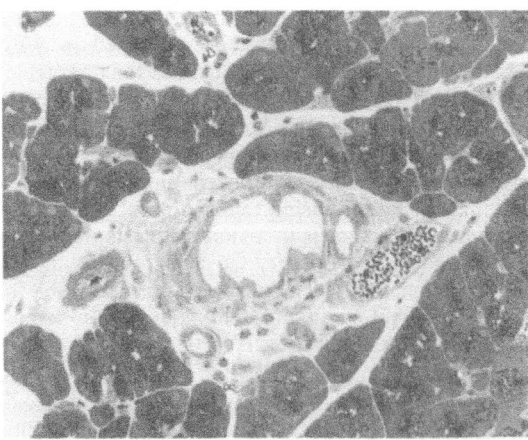

Figure 1. Photomicrograph of epon-embedded pancreatic ducts from a two-month old IFN-γ transgenic mouse. Note several thickened regions around the border of the large duct as a result of cell proliferation. x 400.

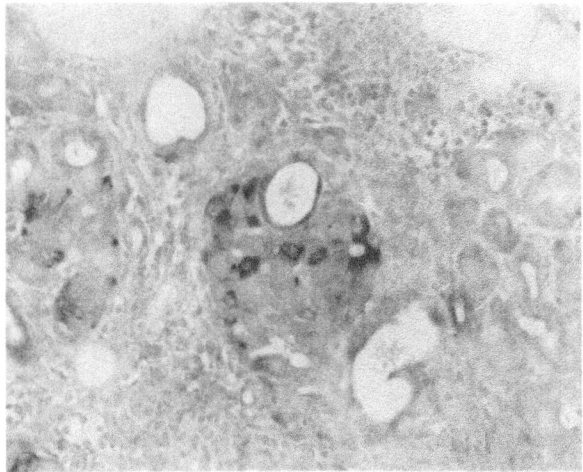

Figure 2. Photomicrograph of a paraffin-embedded section of pancreas from a two-month old IFN-γ transgenic mouse stained with anti-glucagon antibody. A few cells stained positively in this islet-like structure. Note the "islet" is bordering a duct x 400.

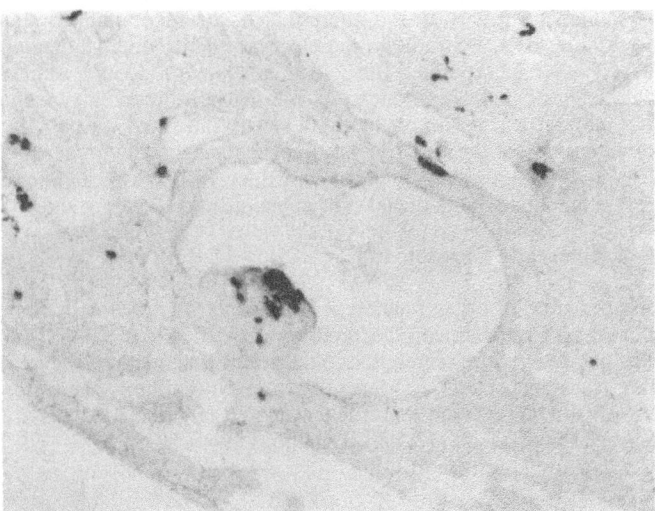

Figure 3. Photomicrograph of a frozen section of pancreas from an eight-month IFN-γ transgenic mouse labeled with anti-insulin antibody. This micrograph shows an islet-like structure grows into the lumen. Note numerous cells in the structure stained strongly with anti-insulin antibody indicating β–cells in nature x 100.

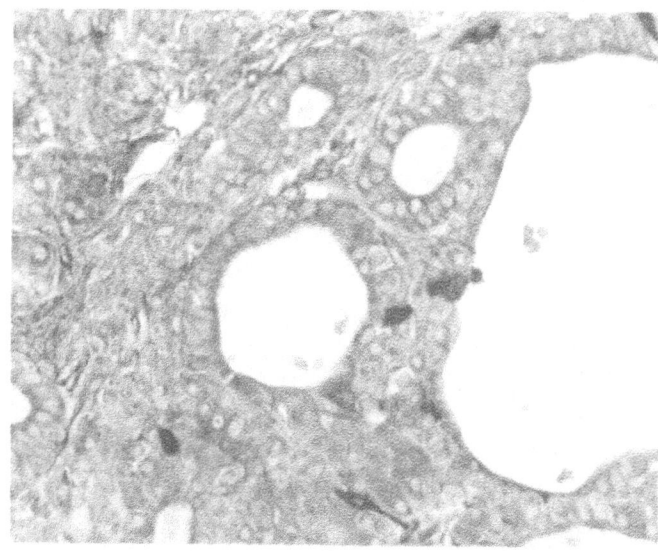

Figure 4. Photomicrograph of a paraffin-embedded section of pancreas from a 80-day old IFN-γ transgenic mouse labeled with anti-somatostatin antibody. Note several ducts are found in this region, suggesting strong proliferative activity of the duct cells. A few somatostatin-containing cells are located nearthe duct epithelial cells x 200.

uridine (BrdU) and revealed by immuno-peroxidase or immunogold methods. The results show very high mitotic activities of the pancreatic duct cells from IFN-γ transgenic mice (Data not shown). Nearly all of the BrdU staining cells reside in the duct wall. Only a few scattered cells stained positively in the interstitial tissue space and no stained cells are detected in the existing islets. Similarly, the electron microscopic studies also reveal that numerous duct cells have incorporated BrdU (data not shown). Double staining of BrdU in conjunction with each of three hormones indicate that all three cell types are capable of replication (data not shown). The results have been confirmed, in part, by the electron microscopic observation that the BrdU incorporated cells also contain dense granules of β-type (data not shown). The results from pancreatic ducts of BALB/C and nonobese diabetes (NOD) mice reveal that none of the ductal cells contain BrdU (Data not shown).

Identification of Pancreatic Hepatocytes

A transdifferentiation of organ phenotype from pancreatic duct cells to hepatocyes has been reported in the rat islets recovering from a copper-deficient diet.[13] Specific antibodies to albumin and alpha-fetoprotein are chosen to determine whether hepatocytes are present in the regenerating transgenic islets. The results from both albumin and alpha-fetoprotein staining experiments have revealed that a few scattered large hepatocytes are found in the interstitial space and the periductal regions (Data not shown).

SUMMARY

We have shown that the pancreatic duct cells of IFN-γ mouse are actively multiplying and that many duct cells differentiate to become endocrine cells. This islet regenerating process closely parallels the islet development during normal organogenesis in the fetus and offers a model for studying the cell lineage relationships of islet cells.[2,3] The subject has received wide interest and intensive research in recent years.[1,5,14-19]

One of the noteworthy results of this study is the finding that duct cells retain the ability to proliferate and to differentiate into islet cells. Under normal conditions, duct cells do not continue to multiply or to differentiate. The results suggest that in the transgenic mice, the progenitor cells of embryonic multipotential duct cells transform into adult cells, but in the presence of appropriate signals or stimuli can resume their multipotential property. The appearance of hepatocytes indicates that while the cell proliferation observed largely results in endocrine cells, other differentiation pathways are occasionally possible. We also detect a few large cells containing albumin and alpha-fetoprotein in the periductal area. Pancreatic hepatocytes have also been observed in the rat after recovery from copper deficiency diet.[13] Thus, the regeneration of islet cells in transgenic mice provides a model system for the study of factors modulating the growth pattern as well as the differentiation pathway.

ACKNOWLEDGEMENTS

We thank Dr. Cheng-ming Chang of the Electron Microscope Labratory, at the Scripps Research Institute, for his generous help with the electron microscopic studies.

REFERENCES

1. P.M. Dubois, Ontogeny of the endocrine pancreas, Horm. Res. 32:53-60 (1989).
2. R.L. Pictet, W.R. Clark, R.H. Williams, and W.J. Rutter, An ultrastructural analysis of the developing embryonic pancreas, Dev Biol. 29:436-67 (1972).
3. R. Picket, and W.J. Rutter, Development of the embryonic endocrine pancreas, In Handbook of Physiology, Sec. 7., D. F. Steiner and M. Frankel, eds.,American Physiological Society, Washington D. C., (1972).
4. I.C. Green, S.E. Seifi, D. Perrin, and L. Howell, Cell replication in the islets of Langerhans of adult rats: effects of frequency, overiectomy and treatment with steroid hormones, J Endocrinol. 88:219-24. (1981)
5. G. Teitelman, S. Alpert, and D. Hanahan, Proliferation, senescence, and neoplastic progression of B cells in hyperplastic pancreatic islets, Cell. 52:97-105 (1988).
6. L. Herberg and D.L. Coleman, Laboratory animals exhibiting obesity and diabetes syndromes, Metabolism. 26:59-99 (1977).
7. D. Hanahan, Heritable formation of pancreatic beta cell tumors in transgenic mice expressing recombinant insulin/simianvirus 40 oncogenes, Nature. 315:115-22 (1985).
8. J.S. Brockenbrough, G.C. Weir, and S. Bonner-Weir, Discordance of exocrine and endocrine growth after 90% pancreatectomy in rats, Diabetes. 37:232-36 (1988).
9. F.E. Smith, K.M. Rosen, L. Villa-Komaroff, G.C. Weir, and S. Bonner-Weir, Enhanced insulin-like growth factor I gene expression in regenerating rat pancreas, Proc Natl Acad Sci USA. 88:6152-56 (1991).
10. L. Rosenberg, this volume.
11. N. Sarvetnick, D. Liggitt, S.L. Pitts, S.E. Hansen, and T.A. Stewart, Insulin-dependent diabetes mellitus induced in transgenic mice by ectopic expression of class II MHC and interferon-gamma, Cell. 52:773-82 (1988).
12. N. Sarvetnick, J. Shizuru, D. Liggitt, L. Martin, B. McIntyre, A. Greggory, T. Parslow, and T. Stewart, Loss of pancreatic islet tolerance induced by B-cell expression of interferon-g, Nature 346:844-47 (1990).
13. M.S. Rao, R.S. Dwivedi, A.V. Yeldandi, V. Subbarao, X. Tan, M.I. Usman, S. Thangada, M.R. Neimali, S. Kumar, S. Scarpelli, and J.K. Reddy, Role of periductal and ductular epithelial cells of the adult rat pancreas in pancreatic hepatocyte lineage: a change in the differentiation commitment, Am J Pathol. 134:1069-86 (1989).
14. G. Tietelman and J.K. Lee, Cell lineage analysis ofpancreatic islet cell development: glucose and insulin cells arise from catecholaminergic precursors present in the pancreatic duct, Dev Biol. 121:454-66 (1987).
15. G. Tietelman, J.K. Lee, and S. Alpert, Cell lineage analysis pancreatic exocrine and endocrine cells, Cell Tissue Res. 250:435-39 (1987).
16. S. Alpert, D. Hanahan, and G. Teitelman, Hybrid insulin genesreveal a developmental lineage for pancreatic endocrine cells and imply a relationship with neurons, Cell 53:295-308 (1988).
17. S. Baekkeskov, H-J Aanstoot, S. Christgau, A. Reetz, M. Solimena, M. Cascalho, F. Folli, H. Richter-Olesen, and P-D Camilli, Identification of the 64K autoantigen in insulin-dependent diabetes as the GABA-synthesizing enzyme glutamic acid decarboxylase, Nature. 347:151-56 (1990).
18. N.M. Le Douarin, On the origin of pancreatic endocrine cells, Cell. 53:169-71 (1988).
19. A. Andersson, On factors that regulate growth of transplanted islets, J Autoimmunity. 3 (Suppl.):131-36 (1990).

DISCUSSION

A. Vinik: Do you think that it would be fair to say that in islet regeneration as opposed to islet restructuring, the net balance will determine whether or not you have diabetes? And is it entirely feasible that we can stimulate islet growth from ducts that could strike out the destructive process of autoimmunity and therefore, be able to help with treating diabetes?

N. Sarvetnick: I think that is true in that I have two lines of mice. One becomes very diabetic and the other one really keeps up more so with the regeneration - I mean the proliferation seems to be higher. In fact, it is the second line that I have been working with more on these regeneration studies. So yes, I think it is possible. However, unless there is immuno-reactive build-up that I've gotten rid of, there is going to be visible inflammatory response that is alright to continue. You could refuel those cells to be replenished and keep the immune response in check by OKT3 antiserum. Their own beta cells are going to be the best ones, because they are compatible.

A. Vinik: Can we bring up another small issue, that maybe, some of the islet people can help us with? Perhaps, the duct of the pancreas is a privileged site for islets. Do we know anything about placing islets within ducts to see whether they are tolerated? And secondly, those of us involved in lumenology - the secretion of hormones into the lumen of the gastrointestinal tract - would be interested in whether the insulin is being delivered by the lumen of the gut as opposed to being delivered in an endocrine or paracrine manner.

N. Sarvetnick: I think those islets would have to become vascular islets in order to grow. Then, I've seen some that are pretty big without an apparent vascular supply. That I do not understand. But I have seen some big islets growing in the middle of ducts, I mean some real hot-dog-sized ones in the duct. The long islets grow along the inside of the duct, so I would think that they would have to become vascularized and why they don't get inflamed - I mean the sort of influx of cells that occurs in the inflammatory response, based on there being a certain kind of vessel around - is beyond my understanding! It may be that for some reason when they become vascularized they don't get the right type of vessels to allow the lymphocytes in. I would think, though, that they would have to be vascularized for the hormones ocurring in the duct to enter the bloodstream.

C. Newgard: Are these islets protected by the duct super islets? Why do you think you are able to correct the hyperglycemia? How many islets are required?

N. Sarvetnick: Well, I just look at the sections, not the whole pancreas. I might see a few of the super islets. I don't know how many are there; we have never actually done any type of morphometry to see if there are 10, or 50.

C. Newgard:	It's remarkable, though, if the diabetes is being controlled.
N. Sarvetnick:	Yes, but see there are always the odd islets that hang around prior to being killed and these could be sufficient to combat hyperglycemia. There could be a significant number in the duct; I didn't show pictures of them but islets between those in the duct and the ones near the duct might be enough to secrete sufficient insulin. That's the only way I could explain why a mouse can be normoglycemic. There are no normal islets.
C. Newgard:	Why don't you just isolate the different islets from the ducts and study them to see if they respond to secretogogues normally?
N. Sarvetnick:	We don't do those physiologic-type studies.
C. Newgard:	In spite of intense controversy about immune privilege, does anyone place islets directly into the central nervous system, i.e., in an immunologically-privileged site?
D. Dafoe	That has been done by, I think the name is Tze, and it is indeed a privileged site.
N. Sarvetnick:	To some extent. Unless antigens leak out of the brain and the brain is a priviledged site. Eventually, you will see immunologic-reactivity. Once the antigens begin to leak out and are detected peripherally and the response in the central nervous system is intact.
A. Vinik:	You referred to Gladys Teitelman's work, because the stage of evolution of her work looks as if you go through a neural phase and show that tyrosine hydroxylase is increased.
N. Sarvetnick:	Well, it's not a real neural phase; it's just that she shows that there are enzymes in the catacholamine pathway that are shared between the primitive gut cells and the brain. In islets you see expression of tyrosine hydroxylase so, at least, according to Teitelman's work that's a different type of cell, not necessarily derived from the neurons.
A. Vinik:	Except that in her recent paper on fetal islets she showed that fetal islets under correct conditions are capable of differentiating into neurons.
N. Sarvetnick:	Right, but there are a lot of different cell types including neurons in islets and I don't know that she has shown in her work, the exact ontogeny of the cells that she is looking at. But it is a nice thought.
A. Vinik:	Do you find neurofibrillary tangles growing out of your islet regeneration model?
N. Sarvetnick:	No, we have not looked. I'm actually going to look, but I have not done so yet. I think that is a nice concept and I was really struck when I saw their work. It is just very hard to say where the neurites are coming from because islets are innervated and you see those cells around, and you can see them if you do a neural stain, certainly, even in a normal islet.
R. Rafaeloff:	In islet cells and neurons tyrosine hydroxylase (TH) is about the same. Do you have any cells that stain for both tyrosine hydroxylase and any of the hormones?

N. Sarvetnick: Oh, you double label the TH and insulin. We haven't done that yet. We are still, right now trying to do BUDR plus TH and the different hormones in which we still can't do the glucagon, and we are trying to do BUDR plus TH to see if hormones, ennzymes, and amines are co-expressed within one cell.

A. Vinik: The reason you may not be getting glucagon right is that you may be seeing precursor glucagon. Carboxyterminal of glucagon in the pancreas may be specifically expressed late. You might have to use an enteroglucagon-type of antiserum or a glicentin-type antiserum to look at the precursor formed early.

N. Sarvetnick: With the polyclonal antibodies, we see plenty of glucagon positive cells budding off the ducts. I'm talking about double labels with BUDR, which is what I would have expected to see - a lot of the cells in the duct double labeling for BUDR plus glucagon. We've seen cells labeling for BUDR plus some somatostatin, not so much double labeling for BUDR plus insulin and glucagon. I actually have the slides amongst these, but I was too embarrassed to show them. The background is very high -I think, due to the acid treatment, so we are sort of trying to determine if we are going by a classical ontogeny or whether there is some sort of shortcut mechanism involved. It will be interesting to see whether or not through this regenerative process the growths are really different, and whether there is a different type of pathway.

TROPHIC STIMULATION OF THE DUCTULAR-ISLET CELL AXIS:
A NEW APPROACH TO THE TREATMENT OF DIABETES

Lawrence Rosenberg, M.D., Ph.D.,[1] and Aaron I. Vinik, M.D., Ph.D.[2]

[1]Montreal General Hospital
 McGill University
 Department of Surgery
 Montreal, Quebec H3G 1A4

[2]Eastern Virginia Medical School
 The Diabetes Institutes
 Norfolk, Virginia 23510

INTRODUCTION

The isolation of insulin in 1922 by Banting and Best laid the foundation for the modern management of diabetes mellitus. While the life expectancy of diabetic patients has been extended, the emergence of secondary complications such as macrovascular disease, retinopathy, neuropathy and nephropathy, is currently responsible for the devastating morbidity and mortality of this disease. Intensive conventional medical therapy has not yet been shown to effectively address these problems and this may relate to an inexact control of the metabolic derangement.

Transplantation of an effective islet cell mass represents a more physiologic approach to therapy. However whole organ pancreas transplantation is far from an ideal solution, and the long-term viability of islet cell allografts appears to be a major unforeseen problem. Therefore, new strategies that seek to reestablish a normal islet cell mass need to be developed.

Adjustments of islet cell number and mass are a means by which an organism may meet changes in the demand for islet hormone production. However in insulin-dependent diabetes the balance is such, that β-cell regeneration is insufficient to overcome the ongoing autoimmune mediated destruction.

The rate of mitosis is quite low in pancreatic β-cells. Consequently the entire complement of β-cells in an adult is established during the neonatal period. This lack of mitotic capacity highlights the "terminal" nature of β-cell differentiation which persists in the adult despite the presence of ductular epithelium, from which the islets are derived embryologically. The factors controlling islet cell neogenesis from ductular epithelium in the adult gland remain unknown and knowledge of their activity may explain the inability of the diabetic to regenerate an adequately functioning islet cell mass.

There are practical reasons, therefore, to elucidate (1) whether islet cells in the adult pancreas retain the capacity to undergo proliferation, (2) whether a pool of precursor cells persists in postnatal life, (3) factors that can induce these cells to undergo endocrine cell differentiation and (4) whether function of newly regenerated islet cells is regulated in a normal manner.

The studies described in this chapter are part of our long-term plan of investigation of the concept that restoration of a functional islet cell mass can be achieved by the induction of pancreatic endocrine cell differentiation from primitive ductal cells. Our primary objective has been to characterize the factors that control the differentiation and growth of pancreatic islet cells, in order to elucidate the potential for eliciting a regenerative response in diabetes. The hypotheses underlying these investigations are enumerated below:

1. The ability of the pancreas to regenerate a functioning islet cell mass is preserved in the post-natal period.
2. Regeneration is mediated by a growth factor(s) that is intrinsic to the gland that is reactivated by cellophane wrapping of the pancreas.
3. This factor, which we have termed "ilotropin," acts directly or indirectly on a stem cell within or, associated with the ductular epithelium to induce endocrine cell differentiation.
4. New islet formation in this model reiterates the normal ontogeny of islet cell development.

DEVELOPMENT OF A MODEL TO STUDY ISLET CELL PROLIFERATION AND DIFFERENTIATION

Choice of Animal

Over the past two decades, the use of the Syrian golden hamster as an experimental animal to study pancreatic regeneration without neoplasia, has increased due to this rodent's response to stimuli that can alter the growth and development of the pancreas and to the very low incidence of spontaneous pancreatic tumors.[1]

Choice of Experimental Model

The models that have been developed to examine the process of islet formation are discussed elsewhere in this monograph. In this chapter we propose to describe the creation of a new model to study islet cell proliferation and differentiation.

In 1982, we developed a method for producing partial obstruction of the hamster pancreatic duct, and noted that this led to new islet formation.[2] The method consisted of wrapping a piece of cellophane tape around the head of the pancreas without duct ligation

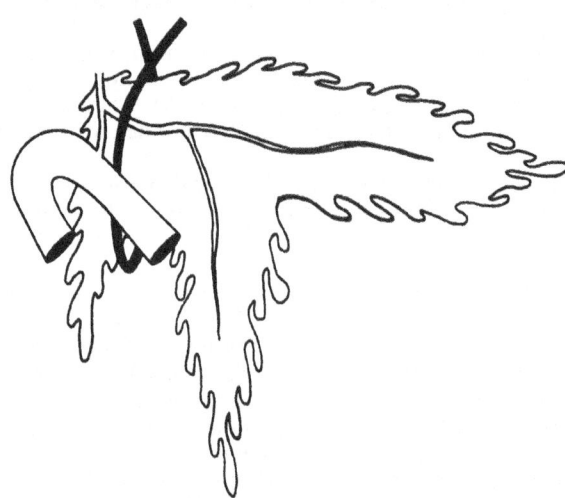

Figure 1. The cellophane wrap model for the induction of cell proliferation and the differentiation in the pancreas. A 2mm wide strip of cellophane tape is placed, under direct vision with the aid of a dissecting microscope, in an avascular plane circumferentially around the head of the pancreas.

per se (Figure 1). The advantage of our model for the induction of islet formation is that proliferative changes can be studied in the absence of diffuse pancreatitis, autoimmune destruction or tissue atrophy, and does not require the addition of chemical agents. As we will discuss in greater detail later in this chapter, the endocrine regeneration induced by cellophane wrapping appears to be primarily a reiteration of the normal ontogeny of the islet from a ductular cell precursor, and not as a result of mitosis of existing β-cells. The trophic effects observed in our model are mediated by a paracrine/autocrine mechanism, and we have extracted from the pancreas a factor that appears to be responsible for the initiation of new islet formation. It is also of importance that our model uses adult animals to study factors that elicit growth potential of cells even when they have reached maturity.

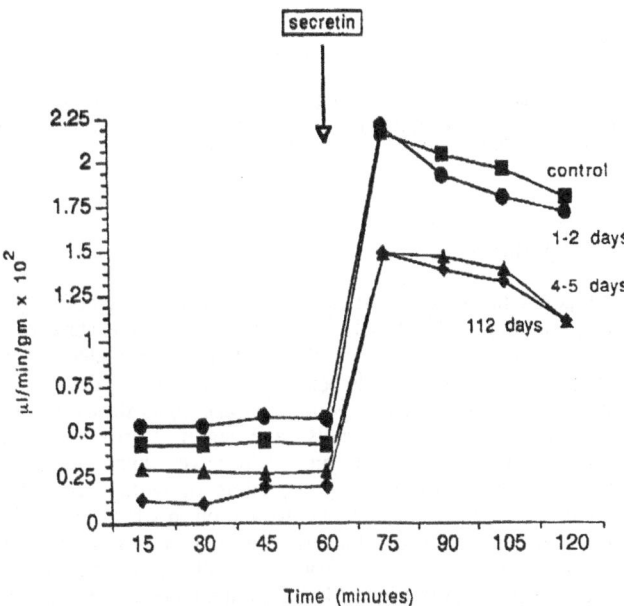

Figure 2. Pancreatic exocrine secretory profile in control hamsters (-B-) and in hamsters on days 1-2 (-J-), 4-5 (-H-) and 112 (-F-) after wrapping. Note that both the basal and secretin stimulated secretion is reduced as early as 48 hours after wrapping and that no further reduction occurs with time.

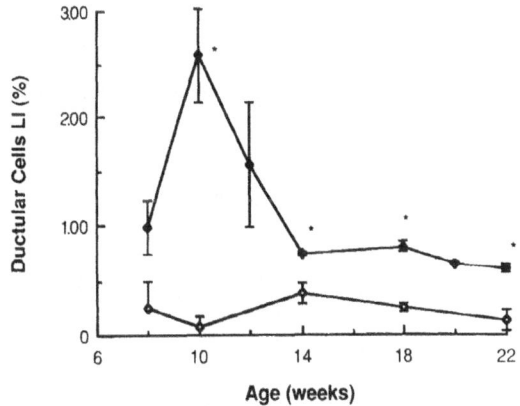

Figure 3. The effect of cellophane wrapping on the incorporation of tritiated thymidine (^{3}H-TdR) into DNA by ductular epithelial cells (-J-), expressed as an index of percentage of cells labelled, in the pancreas of the Syrian golden hamster (n = 4). * p < 0.05.

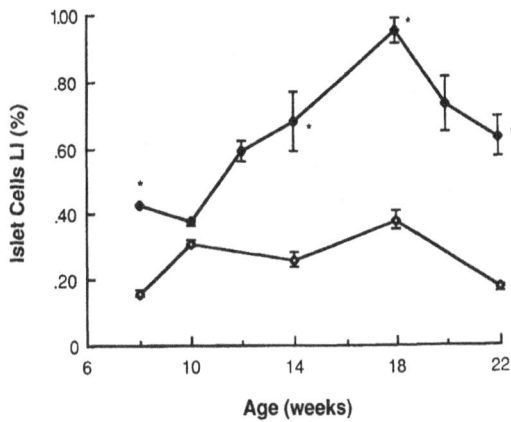

Figure 4. The effect of cellophane wrapping on the initial incorporation of ^{3}H-TdR into DNA by islet cells (-J-), expressed as an index of percentage of cells labelled, in the pancreas of the Syrian golden hamster (n = 4). (o) labelling index for sham-operated control animals (n = 4). * p < 0.05.

The Cellophane Wrap Model

The earliest response to partial obstruction of the pancreas by cellophane wrapping is seen on Day 4-5 after surgery, and consists of ductular dilatation and stasis of secretions. This corresponds with a decrease in both basal and secretin-stimulated pancreatic exocrine secretion (Figure 2), with the lowest levels being reached after 4-5 days.[2-4] At two weeks, proliferation in the ductular epithelial cell population occurs as shown by autoradiographic labeling studies (Figure 3). By Day 21, cells have begun to grow out from the ductular epithelium leading to new islet formation. We have characterized 3 patterns of differentiation by immunohistochemistry: (1) islets in which glucagon, insulin and somatostatin are expressed; (2) foci of new islet formation in which only one islet hormone is expressed, usually either insulin or glucagon, and (3) individual cells in the ductular epithelium staining for glucagon or insulin. By eight weeks, a second wave of proliferation occurs, primarily in the islet cells (Figure 4). Computer-assisted morphometric analysis demonstrated that the induction of new islet formation produced a 2-1/2 -fold increase in the islet cell mass (mean ± SD, expressed as the number of islets/mm^2) from 1.1 ± 0.9 to 2.4 ± 0.8 that was accounted for by the appearance of a new population of small islets (Table 1). These data suggested to us that the new islet cells developed by a process of endocrine differentiation from a precursor cell associated with the ductular epithelium (Figure 5).

Table 1. Observed and Predicted Distribution of Islet Size in Wrapped and Non-wrapped Hamsters.

Islet diameter (μm)	Observed percentage of islet population		Predicted % of Islet population
	Control	Treated	
> 100	63	33	75
< 100	32	67	25
< 48	1	26	5

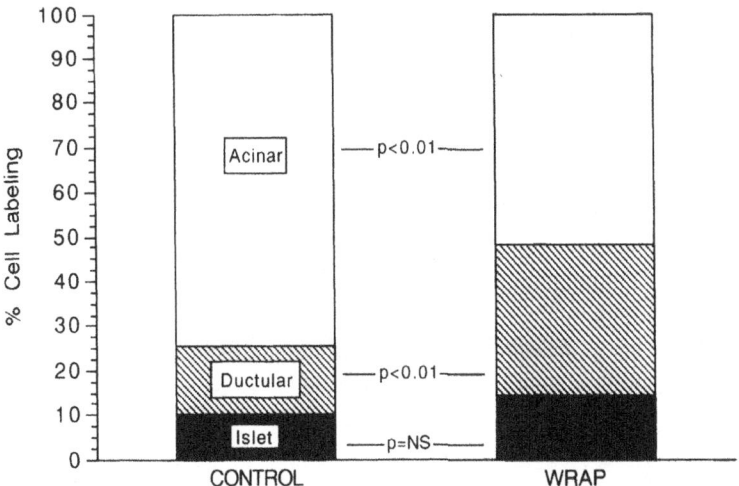

Figure 5. Total ^{3}H-TdR labelling of pancreatic cell compartments 8 weeks after cellophane wrapping (n = 4), compared to age-matched, sham-operated, control animals (n = 4).

In spite of the increased islet cell mass, blood levels of glucose and insulin remain normal after cellophane wrapping of the pancreas of normal animals.[2,3] Moreover, islets that are isolated from the wrapped pancreas of normal animals[5] and perifused in-vitro respond with a normal insulin secretory response to glucose stimulation. These data suggest that even with an increased islet mass, feedback regulation occurs with appropriate adjustment of insulin levels for the prevailing level of glucose. Increased islet mass without apparent increase in insulin levels could concurrently have been due to insulin in the wrapped pancreas being secreted in an altered form. Circulating insulin from non-wrapped and wrapped pancreata were compared by HPLC (Figure 6a and 6b). This analysis suggested that a different molecular species of insulin might indeed be secreted by β-cells in the wrapped pancreas.[5]

To determine whether this insulin was biologically active we undertook to cellophane wrap the pancreases of hamsters rendered diabetic with the β-cell toxin, streptozotocin. Before surgery, the serum glucose(389.0 ± 18.6 mg%) and insulin (33.9 ± 3.8 μU/ml) levels (mean $\pm$ SEM) in unoperated control animals did not differ from those in the animals having the operation (373.2 ± 18.6 mg%; 37.9 ± 3.8 μU/ml) respectively.

After seven weeks, 50% of the operated animals had serum glucose and insulin levels that were normal, compared to only 12% of the unoperated control animals. Islets from normoglycemic operated animals were characterized by increased numbers, including many small islets, positive immunoreactive insulin staining, and minimal vacuolation of cells. Islets from hyperglycemic operated hamsters and from the unoperated control animals were decreased in number and generally larger in size, demonstrated little or no immunoreactive insulin staining and exhibited marked vacuolation of cells.[6,7] From these studies we concluded that cellophane wrapping of the pancreas induced the formation of islets with endocrine cells that are functionally capable of reversing streptozotocin-induced diabetes.

The mechanism by which partial obstruction in our model initiates cell growth, proliferation and differentiation are unknown. To determine if humoral factors are involved, and in particular whether the trophic effect is the result of the local release of a growth factor(s), we studied cellophane wrapping of the hamster pancreas using a parabiotic experimental design.

Pairs of parabiotic hamsters were established and partial duct obstruction produced by wrapping was induced in one parabiont from each pair. At six weeks, the pancreatic gastric lobe weight, DNA, and protein content showed significant increases of 32%, 20% and 28% respectively, over the non-wrapped parabionts (Table 2). Morphometric analysis of the pancreatic splenic lobes demonstrated the presence of new islet formation in the wrapped pancreata with a 100% increase in the number from 0.90 ± 0.50 to 1.8 ± 0.7 islets/mm^2 over

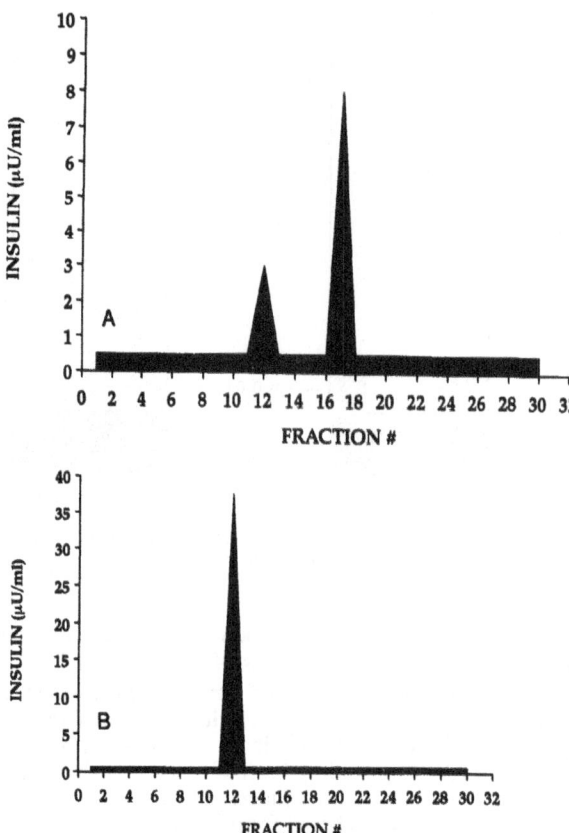

Figure 6. Separation of insulins in non-wrapped (A) and cellophane-wrapped hamsters (B) by reverse-phase HPLC. The data presented represents the mean values for six animals in each group. The chromatography of insulin was performed with fractions collected during in-vitro islet perfusion. A gradient system with two solvents was used. Solvent A consisted of 0.1% tri-fluoroacetic acid in water and solvent B was 0.08% tri-fluoroacetic acid in acetonitril. The column (Vydac C4) was eluted with an initial concentration of solvent B in A+B of 26% to a final concentration of 33% at an incremental rate of 0.1%/min.

Table 2. The Trophic Effect of Cellophane Wrapping of the Pancreas Using a Parabiotic Model.

Parabiont	Tissue Weight (mg)	Tissue Protein (μg)	Tissue DNA	# Islets/mm^2
Non-Wrapped	130 ± 17	21.2 ± 1.9	795 ± 159	0.90 ± 0.50
Wrapped	167 ± 21*	25.4 ± 2.7*	1052 ± 206*	1.80 ± 0.70†

* Significantly ($p < 0.05$) different from non-wrapped
† Significantly ($p < 0.01$) different from non-wrapped

non-wrapped controls. These data suggest that the trophic effects observed in this model of islet cell proliferation and differentiation appear not to be mediated by a humoral mechanism, and control of pancreatic endocrine growth in this model appears to involve paracrine and/or autocrine regulatory mechanisms.[8,9]

As a result of this finding, we prepared extracts of wrapped pancreas and identified one that contained trophic activity that could not be ascribed to known hormones and growth factors. An extract prepared from a non-wrapped pancreas had no such activity.[10] We therefore hypothesized that the trophic activity contained in the tissue extract of wrapped pancreas was due to a potentially novel islet cell growth factor(s). Using a variety of classical protein chemistry techniques, we have identified a soluble polypeptide that we have termed ilotropin. Ilotropin has only been partially characterized as a protein(s) which is trypsin-sensitive, heat stable, acid stable, alcohol precipitable, with an apparent molecular weight in the range of 29-44 kD, and is not sialated. The protein chemistry and purification of ilotropin are the subject of more detailed discussion elsewhere in this text(Pittenger, Rosenberg, Vinik).

We have used an in-vivo bioassay to track the trophic activity of ilotropin at successive stages of purification. Daily injection of a partially purified preparation of ilotropin for 2 days increases pancreatic weight and DNA content by 15% and 40% respectively.[11] After 3 weeks,[12] tritiated thymidine (^{3}H-Tdr) incorporation into ductular and islet cells is increased significantly, and endocrine cell differentiation, comparable to that produced by cellophane wrapping, is observed (Figure 7).

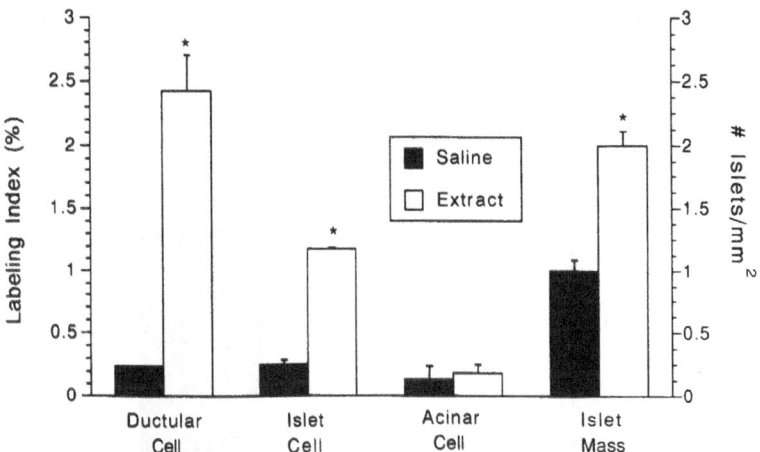

Figure 7. The effect of ilotropin on cell proliferation and islet cell mass in the pancreas. A cell labelling index (LI%) was determined from autoradiograms prepared after 21 days of treatment with the extract. The uptake of ^{3}H-TdR by ductular and islet cells showed a 10- and 6-fold increase over controls. Morphometric analysis demonstrated a 100% increase in the number of islets/mm^2.

In order to directly implicate ilotropin in the trophic effects of wrapping, we treated diabetic hamsters for six weeks with twice daily intraperitoneal injections of ilotropin. Using this regimen, diabetes was stabilized or reversed in 60% of the ilotropin-treated animals, compared to only 10% of saline-treated controls.[13] Extracts of non-wrapped pancreas fare no better than saline-treated and at most induce remission in 12% of animals. The successful treatment of diabetes in this setting was achieved by the induction of a new population of insulin producing β–cells (Figures 8 and 9) .

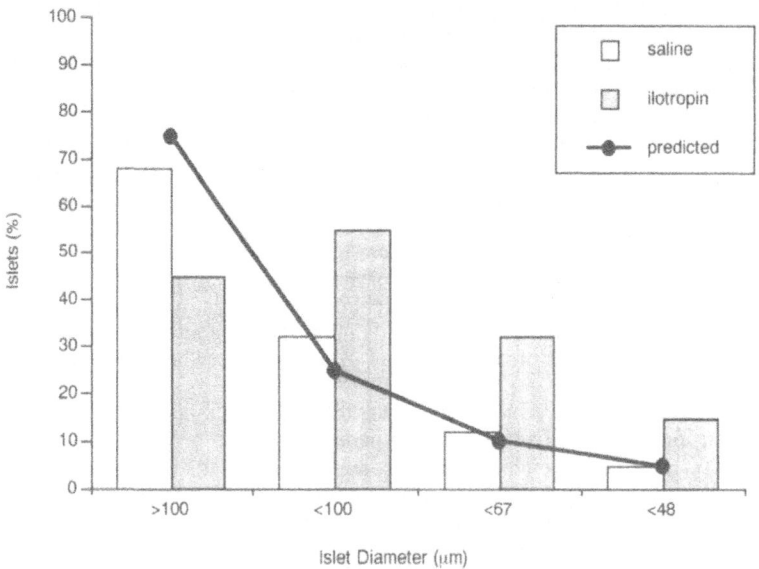

Figure 8. Observed and predicted distribution of islet size in ilotropin treated and saline control animals. The population distribution of islet size in the control animals corresponded to the predicted values for the normal hamster pancreas. In the ilotropin treated animals, in comparison to the control group, an initial significant shift in the distribution of islet size (p < 0.01) that corresponded to the appearance of a new population of small islets was demonstrated. Islets do however, grow to be larger than normal and then appear to return to normal size.

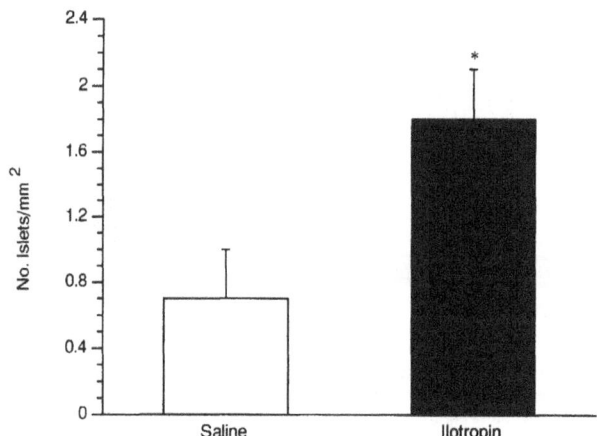

Figure 9. Islet cell mass (# islets/mm^2) in hamsters treated for 7 weeks with either ilotropin or saline. The islet cell mass in the normoglycemic, ilotropin-treated, animals was increased significantly (p < 0.01) when compared to both saline controls and the ilotropin-treated animals that remained hyperglycemic (not shown), i.e., hyperglycemia per se was an insufficient stimulus to generate a growth response.

Questions have arisen as to the species specificity of the effects. For this reason we examined the effects of wrapping in different species for regeneration. The effects of cellophane wrapping of the pancreas (Figures 10 and 11) can also be induced in the pancreas of the cat and rat. Therefore the trophic effects of partial duct obstruction are not species specific, but may presumably be generalized to other large mammals, possibly even including man.

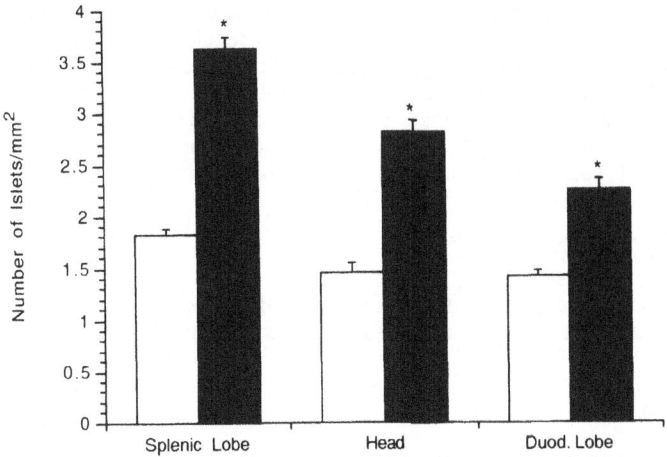

Figure 10. The effect of cellophane wrapping (-■-) on the islet cell mass in the cat pancreas compared to non-wrapped controls (-□-). * (p < 0.01). Note that the effect is not localized only to the lobe wrapped.

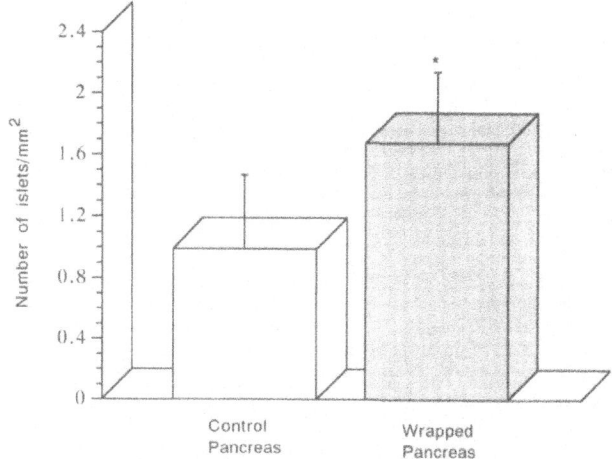

Figure 11. The effect of cellophane wrapping on the islet cell mass in the rat pancreas. * (p < 0.01).

Over 50 years ago, the pancreatic exocrine outflow in diabetic children was partially obstructed in a manner similar to the technique of cellophane wrapping described here. This surgical manipulation reportedly produced an increase in 'sugar tolerance' compatible with our observation in lower mammals,[14,15] but we can only speculate upon whether the apparent improvement in glucose homeostasis was due to the regeneration of a new β-cell population.

SUMMARY

We have established a model in which cellophane wrapping induces reiteration of the normal ontogeny of β-cell differentiation from ductal tissue. The secretion of insulin is physiologic and coordinated to the needs of the animal. Streptozotocin-induced diabetes in hamsters can be "cured" at least 1/2 the time. There appears to be activation of growth factor(s) within the pancreas acting in an autocrine, paracrine or juxtacrine manner to induce ductal cell proliferation and differentiation into functioning β-cells. Given the results of our studies to date, it does not seem premature to envisage new approaches to the treatment of diabetes mellitus. Identification of the factor(s) which regulate islet cell proliferation and differentiation in our model may permit islets to be grown in culture. This concept could be extended to induce endocrine cell differentiation in-vitro as well. Furthermore, islet cell growth factors could be used to provide "trophic support" to islet transplants as a means of maintaining graft viability. There may also be greater scope for gene therapy when the growth factor(s) has been isolated, purified, sequenced and cloned.

ACKNOWLEDGEMENTS

This work was supported by a grant from the National Cancer Institute #1R01CA5464101, Medical Research Council of Canada #MA-10648, and Canadian Diabetes Association.

REFERENCES

1. D.S. Longnecker, Experimental models of exocrine pancreatic tumors, *in:* "The Exocrine Pancreas: Biology, Pathobiology and Diseases," V.L.W. Go, et al., eds., Raven Press, New York (1986).
2. L. Rosenberg, R.A. Brown, and W.P. Duguid, A new model for the development of duct epithelial hyperplasia and the initiation of nesidioblastosis, J Surg Res. 35:63 (1983).
3. L. Rosenberg, Cell proliferation in the pancreas of the Syrian golden hamster. PhD Thesis. Montreal, Quebec, McGill University (1984).
4. L. Rosenberg, W.P. Duguid, and A.I. Vinik, The effect of cellophane wrapping of the pancreas in the Syrian golden hamster: Autoradiographic observations, Pancreas. 4:31-37 (1989).
5. L. Rosenberg and A.I. Vinik, Induction of endocrine cell differentiation- a new approach to the management of diabetes, J Clin Lab Med. 114:75-83 (1989).
6. L. Rosenberg, W.P. Duguid, R.A. Brown, and A.I. Vinik, Induction of islet cell proliferation will reverse diabetes in the Syrian golden hamster, Diabetes. 37:334 (1988).
7. L. Rosenberg, W.P. Duguid, and R.A. Brown, Effect of experimental nesidioblastosis on streptozotocin-induced diabetes, Surg Forum. 34:48-51 (1983).
8. L. Rosenberg and A.I. Vinik, Regulation of pancreatic islet growth and differentiation - Evidence for paracrine and/or autocrine growth factor(s), Clin Res. 38:271A (1990).
9. L. Rosenberg, W.P. Duguid, M. Kahlenberg, and A.I. Vinik, Paracrine/autocrine regulation of pancreatic islet cell proliferation and differentiation in the hamster. Studies using parabiosis. (submitted for publication)
10. L. Rosenberg, D. Thomas, D. Dafoe, et al, Stimulation of pancreatic growth by a cytosol extract derived from the cellophane wrapped pancreas, Surg Forum. 37:168 (1986).
11. L. Rosenberg, D. Clas, and W.P. Duguid, Trophic stimulation of the ductular-islet cell axis: A new approach to the treatment of diabetes, Surgery. 108:191-97 (1990).
12. D. Clas, L. Rosenberg, W.P. Duguid, and E. Malashenko, Islet cell differentiation and proliferation induced by a pancreatic cytosol extract, Surgical Forum. 39:620-24 (1988).
13. L. Rosenberg, W.P. Duguid, M. Healy, D. Clas, and A.I. Vinik, Reversal of diabetes by the induction of islet cell neogenesis, Transplant Proc. (in press).
14. G. de Takats and R.M. Wilder, Isolation of tail of pancreas in a diabetic child, JAMA, 93:606 (1929).
15. G. de Takats and F.P. Cuthbert, Surgical attempts at increasing sugar tolerance, Arch Surg. 68:750 (1933).

DISCUSSION

C. Newgard: Did you find any difference in islet distribution in animals that have completely recovered from normal glycemia versus those that haven't - did you look at that?

L. Rosenberg: Yes, the animals that received ilotropin that did not revert to normal glycemia had either an islet distribution that was intermediate between these two or one that was fairly identical to the control situation. There was only one, as I recall, one ilotropin-treated animal that really had a blood sugar above 22.2; there were three with intermediate blood sugars; and four with what we considered a normal blood sugar, so all of these animals had at least a distribution that approximated the control group and these were somewhat intermediate.

C. Newgard: Does that not surprise you? I would have thought that one would potentially explain that the failure to return to normal glycemia is that, maybe, you have all small islets and that you haven't gotten the full regeneration, if that's what you want to call it, in those that have returned to normal glycemia. You're not surprised that you have a point that would be a normal spectrum size?

L. Rosenberg: Well, it may just be that we didn't wait long enough.

A. Vinik: I think you're on to it because in the earlier experiments, what has been shown, is that the fate of islets is time coordinated. They go through this initial phase as small, intermediate, islets and then become larger than normal, then assume the adult size. It depends on where in time you catch them. I think the single point experiment doesn't give you the whole answer as to what the islet is really doing.

C. Newgard: Can you evoke the same response by wrapping the pancreas in other species of animals? At the same order of magnitude?

L. Rosenberg: Yes, we have done it in cats, and in rats. We haven't repeated all of these studies in those species, but the initial cellophane-wrap experiment did demonstrate that this is not a species-specific phenomenon.

C. Newgard: The reason I ask the question is that the Syrian hamster has one of the most extraordinarily sensitive neuroendocrine systems around and is an exquisitely photo-periodically driven animal, so that there may be an enhancement of the kind of effect you see in this particular species. I would like to see this work in sub-human primates now.

L. Rosenberg:	Yes, I would too.
A. Vinik:	You know what they say . . . "from rats to cats to chimpanzees." We're getting there.
L. Rosenberg:	Actually, this is the type of response I got last year. As I was explaining to Susan Bonner-Weir there are a series of publications in Experimental Medicine, by deTakats, from 1927-1932, which report a duct ligation procedure very similar to this in three diabetic children. At that time of poor technology there was not a very good understanding of diabetes. It was reported in this series of articles that each of these children had an improvement of glucose tolerance. Maybe the process occurs in humans, too.
C. Newgard:	Your allusion to the characterization of the trophic influences I think is very, very critical and I am reminded of the lack and the ignorance, the lack of thinking about this in this huge phenomonology that we call neurografting for Parkinsonism and autografting with the adrenal medulla. And that neurosurgeons weren't really thinking much about the trophic influence, as much as plunking it down into the head of the caudate and hoping it would undergo phenotypic differentiation back into neurons. So I applaud you, I think that this is very exciting.
C. Newgard:	To follow up on that, would you anticipate then that ilotropin as you now have it, and I guess we will hear more about it, would be more effective on pancreas fragments as opposed to isolated islets? Do you think you need the ductal cells to get the effects of the material that you are isolating?
L. Rosenberg:	First, we are not sure where the material comes from. We are not even sure what cells are the target.
C. Newgard:	So there is no direct evidence, or maybe there will be shortly, that isolated islets respond to this material?
L. Rosenberg:	You won't hear about that today.
C. Newgard:	Is it a secret?
L. Rosenberg:	No it's not a secret, we do have preliminary data which indicates that isolated islets were responsive.
C. Newgard:	That's very nice. A different question, just real quick. When you tie off and you get this response, what happens to glucose homeostasis in the normal animal?
L. Rosenberg:	We've measured blood glucose in the cellophane-wrapped animals and it's normal. So we recently measured total glandular content of hormones. We haven't got the data back for the other hormones, but the amount of insulin per cell seems to be reduced.
C. Newgard:	So there are more islets?
L. Rosenberg:	Yes, there are more islets.
C. Newgard:	But is there the same amount of insulin?

L. Rosenberg: There is the same amount of insulin - very preliminary data. But the amount of insulin per cell seems to be less.

C. Newgard: So the glucose challenge you would anticipate, would be normal in the wrapped animal?

L. Rosenberg: I would think so.

A. Vinik: It is important to recognize that the animal is not challenged by hyperglycemia. And it's only when it is called on to do that, that it responds.

B. Glaser: How often did the animals that were injected with the substance develop hyperplasia? Did their glucose stay stable the entire time while they were getting injected with the material?

C. Newgard: Yes, it's kind of a take off again of the invitro effect. The fact is that the parabiosis experiments may suggest that it is not apparent that you see distal effects of a humeral type, and yet when you inject this material, you are seeing an effect. This suggests that you are administering large amounts, which, if you had some way of delivering locally would probably be much, much more potent than you would assess by this *in vivo* technique. Have you tried alternate means of maybe local delivery or direct delivery?

L. Rosenberg: No we haven't. You are quite correct about the possibility that there may be an hormonal effect.

A. Vinik: We would like to get the purified product. We have no idea of what it's actual potency is to be able to start delivering it in appropriate amounts.

S. Bonner-Weir: I'm a little confused - if you are finding it and extracting it at 10 days (I assume that is 10 days) and then you are injecting it for 3 days, then immediately after that you are asserting that you are seeing the peak in ducts, that doesn't make sense.

L. Rosenberg: No, we are seeing it in 3 weeks, not 3 days. The biochemical data on changes in protein and DNA content is after 3 days. The 3H-TdR labeling experiments are after 3 weeks.

S. Bonner-Weir: In the ducts?

L. Rosenberg: Yes, in the ducts.

S. Bonner-Weir: So you are putting it in and then 3 weeks later it shows up in the ducts and 4 weeks after that it shows up in the islet?

L. Rosenberg: No, these studies were not done sequentially, that particular site was sampled at just one point in time at 3 weeks.

A. Vinik: I know we are confusing issues here. Susan, I would like to explain that what Lawrence is saying is that with the injection of the extract used here, changes in pancreatic weight occur very quickly. But, the 3H-TdR uptake into the ducts occurs 3 weeks after the first injection. Unlike your experiments, this turnover is a slower turnover.

S. Bonner-Weir:	But this is when you've done the wrapping or when you've done the injection?
L. Rosenberg:	After the wrapping, the peak of ductular cell labeling is approximately 2 weeks later.
S. Bonner-Weir:	And then the islet is 4 weeks after that?
L. Rosenberg:	That's right.
C. Newgard:	That is recapitulated with your drug treatment?
L. Rosenberg:	This may be so, but we cannot tell for sure because with drug treatment we only looked at the islet markers at one time point.
C. Newgard:	So both are represented? That is, the islets, and ducts respond to both wrapping and injection of the extract? That was my question earlier.
S. Bonner-Weir:	And at that point in time when you did your sampling, were they both represented?
L. Rosenberg:	At the point of sampling, they were significantly greater than the saline injected controls, but if you remember at that point of time in the wrapping experiment, the islet labeling was already on the way up.
J. Nielsen:	Will the nesidioblastosis continue with time? I mean it's probably considered a sort of pathological state or what if they eventually develop a tumor or hypoglycemia?
L. Rosenberg:	I've looked at it up to approximately 15 weeks and the animals were perfectly normal in glucose homeostasis.
J. Nielsen:	And if you remove the cellophane?
L. Rosenberg:	You can't.
N. Sarvetnick:	Have you ever tried wrapping a NOD mouse? That would be more similar to wrapping a human type 1. Presumably, whatever the inflammatory response would be, it would remain constant - but would just provide more target. I'm not saying that anything like this isn't feasible. The perfect combination would be to show that regeneration occurs with ongoing destruction.
L. Rosenberg:	That's something that we've actually started to do. We plan to continue that line of research.
N. Sarvetnick:	You have one mouse already injected?
L. Rosenberg:	Ok, we've already injected ilotropin into the NOD mouse and have seen minor chemical changes in pre-diabetic animals.
N. Sarvetnick:	But what you haven't done is follow them for a long time?
L. Rosenberg:	To see if they get diabetic?
A. Vinik:	Right.
L. Rosenberg:	Well, they probably will.

A. Vinik: The whole idea then would be that the balance between the destruction and our ability to cause regeneration determines the presence or absence of diabetes. That's what Laurence's work is concerned with.

SECTION THREE

INDUCTION OF CELL GROWTH
AND MECHANISMS

EXPRESSION OF INSULIN-LIKE GROWTH FACTORS (IGFs) AND THEIR BINDING PROTEINS (IGF BPs) DURING PANCREATIC DEVELOPMENT IN RAT, AND MODULATION OF IGF ACTIONS ON RAT ISLET DNA SYNTHESIS BY IGF BPs

David J. Hill, Ph.D.,[1] Joanna Hogg, Ph.D.[2]

[1]MRC Group in Fetal and Neonatal Health and Development
Department of Physiology
University of Western Ontario

[2]Lawson Research Institute
St. Joseph's Health Centre
London, Ontario, N6A 4V2, Canada

INTRODUCTION

Growth of pancreatic β-cells is an essential feature of fetal development in order to maintain insulin needs. This is particularly relevant to the growth of the mammalian fetus where there is an ever-increasing demand for insulin both to facilitate the metabolic processes of growth, and to act as a peptide growth factor.[1] An increase in β cell mass may be derived not only from β-cell replication but from the recruitment and maturation of undifferentiated β-cell precursors. In the rat fetus the cellular area staining positively for insulin by immunohistochemistry increases two-fold within two days of the end of gestation. However, only 20% of this increase can be accounted for by the proliferation rate of existing β-cells.[2] The maturation of precursor cells is supported by the observation that DNA synthesis in cells next to growing islets proceeds at a faster rate than in the islets themselves. Similarly, the newborn rat, made diabetic with streptozotocin, exhibits serious β-cell destruction, but at 14 days after birth demonstrates normo-glycemia with considerable mitotic activity being apparent in the non-endocrine cells and the duct epithelium of the pancreas.[3] While metabolic and nutritional control of β cell hyperplasia is well documented,[4] there is a growing cohort of reports that suggest that an endogenous production of growth factors including insulin-like growth factor (IGF)-I and -II may also contribute to the process.[5-9]

Insulin-like growth factors are synthesized and are present within pancreatic endocrine tissue, and have been localized predominantly to β-cells. In human fetal pancreas obtained in early second trimester, duct and islet cells stain positively immunohistochemically with an antiserum that recognizes predominantly IGF-II.[10] A similar pattern of staining is seen for IGF-binding proteins (BPs)-1 and -2.[11,12] IGF immunoreactivity is also present in human fetal pancreas explants following tissue culture[13] and by the staining of adjacent sections of islets for IGFs, insulin, glucagon and somatostatin the IGF can be localized to the β-cell population. The pancreas appears to actively synthesize both IGF-I and -II. Messenger

RNAs encoding both peptides have been identified by Northern blot hybridization in intact human fetal pancreas with approximately 100 times more mRNA for IGF-II than IGF -I.[14]

Several studies have reported the release of immunoassayable IGF peptides from isolated rat islets of Langerhans.[15-17] Schaufmann et al[17] demonstrated that IGF-I present in fetal rat islets was physicochemically similar to that in blood, and was a product of *de novo* synthesis. Evidence that IGFs exert a paracrine/autocrine action during β cell hyperplasia is provided by the findings that: a) exogenous IGF-I or -II are mitogenic for rat islets *in vitro*;[15,18,19] b) exogenous IGF-I stimulates an increase in DNA content in cultured human fetal pancreatic islets,[20] and c) adult rat islets contain type-1 IGF receptors on both A and β-cell populations.[21] Other growth factors may also contribute to β-cell hyperplasia. Swenne et al[18] showed that platelet-derived growth factor (PDGF) stimulates DNA replication in fetal rat islets and, using a monoclonal antibody against hIGF I, indicated that this action was independent of IGF I release. When PDGF and IGF-I were present together their effects were additive. This is consistent with the findings that for other cell types PDGF often acts as a competence factor at the G_0/G_1 interface of the cell cycle, while IGF-I acts as a progression factor in later G_1.[22] Epidermal growth factor (EGF) was reported to stimulate (pro)-insulin biosynthesis and DNA synthesis in isolated adult rat islets.[23] Each of these growth factors are only effective mitogens in the presence of optimal concentrations of glucose. This suggests that glucose, and possibly other nutrients, are the primary stimuli to β-cell proliferation, and that this response can be modulated by polypeptide growth factors.

This report documents a number of studies by us into the expression and release of IGF-I and -II by intact rat pancreas, and by isolated fetal rat islets of Langerhans. In view of the ability of specific IGF binding proteins (IGF BPs) to modulate IGF bioactivity on other cell types[24] we have also considered the contribution of IGF BPs to the control of β-cell hyperplasia.

METHODS

Northern Blot and *in situ* Hybridization

Fetal Wistar rats were killed on days 18, 20 and 22 of gestation and postnatal rats between days 1 and 35 following birth. Pancreas was immediately removed, frozen in liquid nitrogen and stored at -70º C. Tissue was homogenized in 4 M guanidine thiocyanate and total RNA was separated by centrifugation over a cushion of 5.7 M cesium chloride. Total RNA (20 - 30 μg) was denatured for 15 min. at 65º C in 6% deionized formaldehyde and 50 % deionized formamide in 1 x hybridization buffer (20 mM morpholinopropane-sulfonic acid, 5 mM sodium acetate, 5 mM EDTA; pH 7.0) and size fractionated on 1% agarose gels containing 6% deionized formaldehyde. The RNAs were then transferred to Zetaprobe nylon membranes and pre-hybridized for 2 h. with hybridization buffer containing 1 x SSPE (150 mM NaCl, 10 mM sodium phosphate, 1 mM EDTA), 7% SDS, 100 μg/ml salmon sperm DNA and 50% deionized formamide. Hybridization was performed at 42º C overnight with 2 x 10⁶ c.p.m. labelled cDNA probes. After hybridization, blots were washed with 1 x standard citrate saline at 42º C and developed by autoradiography. The following cDNA probes were used: rat IGF-I (gift from Dr. L. Murphy, University of Manitoba), mouse IGF-II (gift from Dr. G. Bell, University of Chicago), and rat IGF BP-1 and BP-2 (gifts from Dr. M. Rechler, National Institutes of Health). Probes were labelled with a ^{32}P dCTP using a Pharmacia random priming oligolabelling kit.

For *in situ* hybridization tissues were fixed in 4% paraformaldehyde/0.2% glutaraldehyde in 70 mM phosphate buffer (pH 7.0) at 4º C overnight. After washing, tissues were embedded in paraffin and 5 μm sections prepared and mounted on polylysine-coated slides. Sense and anti-sense cRNA probes were transcribed from cDNAs in the presence of ^{35}S-UTP with an appropriate specific RNA polymerase (T3 or T7) using the PROMEGA Riboprobe Gemini System, and were hybridized with tissue sections at 50º C for 24 h. (2 x 10⁶ c.p.m. per slide). Hybridization buffer contained 50% deionised formamide, 10% dextran sulfate, 6 x SSC, 2 x Denhardts, 50 mM Tris-HCl (pH 7.0) containing 50 mM EDTA, denatured salmon sperm DNA (0.1 mg/ml) and yeast transfer RNA (0.1 mg/ml). Following hybridization, sections were washed for 1 h. in 2 x SSC at room temperature, for 2

h. in 2 x SSC at 50º C, and for 10 min. in 0.1 x SSC at room temperature, and dehydrated in ethanol. Slides were dipped in NTB-3 photoemulsion, air-dried and exposed in sealed boxes for 7 days at 4º C. After developing, sections were counterstained with hematoxylin and eosin and the hybridization signal with anti-sense cRNA observed using dark field microscopy. As controls for non-specific hybridization, the hybridizations were performed on parallel sections using a) sense probes, and b) anti-sense probes on sections previously incubated with RNAase.

Islet Cell Culture

Fetuses were killed on day 22 of gestation, the pancreas was removed and the islets isolated by a modification of the technique of Hellerstrom et al.[25] Briefly, pancreata were finely chopped and incubated with Hank's buffered salt solution containing 2 mg/ml collagenase (Type V) for 3-5 min. in a shaking water bath at 37º C. The washed digest was resuspended in RPMI 1640 (pH 7.4) containing 11.1 mM glucose and 25 mM HEPES buffer, 10% fetal calf serum and antibiotics. The digest was distributed onto tissue culture-grade plastic petri dishes and incubated at 37º C for 5 days in a humidified atmosphere of 5% CO_2 in air. Growth medium was changed daily. Following five days the islets were detached from the dish by pipette and harvested by hand. Islets were transferred to non-tissue culture grade plastic dishes and cultured free-floating in RPMI 1640 supplemented with 0.7-16.7 mM glucose, 1% fetal calf serum and increasing concentrations of recombinant h IGF-I or -II, hIGF BP-1 or bovine IGF BP-2 (gift of Dr. D. Clemmons, University of North Carolina), or IGFs and IGF BPs in combination for 48 h. Medium was collected for estimation of insulin, IGF-I and IGF-II content by radioimmunoassays, and the presence of IGF BPs using ligand Western blot or immuno-blot. To assess DNA synthetic rate, ^{3}H-thymidine (1uCi/ml) was added for the final 24 h of culture. Islets were harvested, washed and disrupted ultrasonically, and DNA precipitated in 5% ice-cold trichloroacetic acid. The precipitate was collected on a glass-fiber disk and the incorporated radiolabel quantified by liquid scintillation counting. The incorporation of ^{3}H-thymidine into DNA was expressed per μg cell DNA determined by a fluorometric technique.[1] The number of islet cells demonstrating nuclear labelling for ^{3}H-thymidine was determined by pelleting the islets in agar following incubation and fixation in paraformaldehyde/glutaraldehyde. Three μm sections were prepared and exposed to NTB-3 photoemulsion for autoradiography. Sections of islets were also examined for the presence of IGF-I and -II, for IGF BP-2 and for insulin by immunocytochemistry using the avidin-biotin peroxidase technique as described previously.[10] A rabbit anti-human IGF-I antiserum recognizing both IGF-I and -II was provided by Dr. D. Morrell, Institute of Child Health, London; while antiserum against bovine IGF BP-2 was a gift from Dr. D. Clemmons, University of North Carolina. Guinea pig anti-insulin antibody (IDS, Washington. U.K.) was used and all antisera were used at a 1:1000 final dilution. Color was generated with diaminobenzidine and sections counter-stained with hematoxylin and eosin. Controls included pre-incubation of the primary antiserum with excess homologous ligand, substitution with non-immune serum and the omission of the secondary antiserum.

IGF and Insulin Radioimmunoassay

Insulin-like growth factor-I and -II in islet-conditioned media were measured by specific radioimmunoassays as described previously.[25,26] Conditioned media were first extracted by reverse phase chromatography on C18 silica gel mini-columns to separate IGFs from IGF BPs which would otherwise interfere with the radioimmunoassays. The method was as described previously[25] and yielded a reproducible recovery of 55 ± 5% IGF-I and 61 ± 5% IGF-II. Results are corrected for recovery. Insulin was measured by specific radioimmunoassay using a rat insulin standard.

Detection of IGF BPs

Species of IGF BPs released into islet-conditioned medium were characterized with respect to molecular size using a ligand Western blot method described previously.[27] Briefly, conditioned medium (50 ul) was loaded onto an 8% SDS-polyacrylamide gel under non-reducing conditions. Following separation proteins were transferred to 0.2 um nitrocellulose membranes using an electrophoretic blotting apparatus before overnight incubation of the membrane with 400,000 c.p.m. ^{125}I-labelled IGF-II. Following incubation the membranes were washed thoroughly and developed by autoradiography. To identify IGF BP-2 on nitrocellulose filters a modified immuno-blot technique was used as described by Hill et al.[28] The primary antiserum was rabbit anti-bovine IGF BP-2 (1:1000 final dilution) and the avidin-biotin peroxidase technique was used as described above.

RESULTS

Northern hybridization analysis revealed four distinct IGF-II mRNA transcripts to be present in rat pancreas of 1.2, 2.2, 3.9 and 4.8 Kb respectively. IGF-II mRNA abundance was greatest at 18 days gestation and declined over late-gestation and the perinatal period. It was no longer detectable after 14 days postnatal life. Multiple transcripts of IGF-I mRNA were also detected in rat pancreas of 0.7, 1.8, 5.2 and 7.8 Kb respectively. In contrast to IGF-II, the levels of IGF-I mRNA were low but detectable in fetal life and increased in abundance following 14 days postnatal life. When examined by *in situ* hybridization the mRNA encoding IGF-II was found to be distributed throughout the pancreatic, mesenchyme, exocrine tissue and islets. This distribution did not change with age, although the intensity of the hybridization signal was decreased in pancreases from post-natal animals. In the perinatal rat IGF-I mRNA was distributed throughout the pancreatic tissues but following weaning was found only in the exocrine pancreas with no hybridization associated with islet cells.

Messenger RNA encoding IGF BP-1 was not detectable in fetal rat pancreas by Northern hybridization, but a single 1.8 Kb transcript appeared by day 14 of postnatal life, was maximal on day 21 and was of lower abundance in the adult. A single transcript of IGF BP-2 mRNA of 1.6 Kb was detectable at relatively low levels in the fetal pancreas but increased in abundance at 14 and 21 days postnatal life. Levels of IGF BP-2 mRNA were relatively lower in the adult pancreas than at weaning. *In situ* hybridization revealed that both IGF BP-1 and BP-2 mRNAs were contained within the mesenchyme, exocrine tissue and islets of the pancreas and this distribution did not change over the age range at which signals were detectable.

When isolated fetal rat islets of Langerhans were examined by immunocytochemistry, most islets appeared as discrete balls of cells in which almost every cell stained positively for insulin. A minority of islets contained immuno-negative cells with morphology similar to β-cells. After hybridization with an IGF-II cDNA, a single mRNA transcript of 1.8 Kb was detectable by Northern hybridization in RNA isolated from batches of approximately 2000 islets. Using these amounts of islets, hybridization signals for IGF-I, IGF BP-1 and BP-2 could not be detected. However, immunocytochemistry using an antibody which detected both IGF-I and -II revealed that almost every cell making up fetal rat islets contained IGF peptides following culture. Similarly, almost every cell in these structures stained positively for the presence of IGF BP-2.

When isolated fetal rat islets were incubated in medium containing increasing concentrations of glucose between 2.7 mM and 16.7 mM the release of radioimmunoassayable insulin increased with glucose availability with a maximum release in the presence of 8.7 mM glucose (2.7 mM glucose, 2.6 ± 0.4 nM insulin/μg DNA/24 h; 8.7 mM, 6.0 ± 0.6 nM/μg/24 h; 16.7 mM, 5.7 ± 0.4 nM/μg/24 h; mean $\pm$ s.e.m., n = 4). The DNA synthetic rate of islets was also estimated in response to an increasing availability of glucose. The incorporation of ^{3}H-thymidine into DNA also increased with increasing glucose concentrations showing a maximal response at 8.7 mM glucose (2.7 mM glucose, 4.2 ± 0.2 d.p.m.x10^{-3}/10 islets/24 h; 5.6 mM, 6.8 ± 0.3 d.p.mx10^{-3}/10 islets/24 h; 8.7 mM, 7.5 ± 0.3 d.p.m.x10^{-3}/10 islets/24 h; 11.2 mM, 5.8 ± 0.3 d.p.m.x10^{-3}/10 islets/24 h; mean $\pm$ s.e.m., n = 4). When the DNA synthetic rate was determined by autoradiography the nuclear labelling index in the presence of 2.7 mM glucose was 12%, and in the presence of 8.7 mM glucose was 22%. Only the nuclei of cells which were immunohistochemically positive for insulin were seen to label with ^{3}H-thymidine.

Under basal culture conditions with 2.7 mM glucose both IGF-I and -II were detected by radioimmunoassays in the medium conditioned by isolated fetal rat islets, the release of IGF-II being approximately twice that of IGF-I (IGF-I, 0.1 ± 0.3 nM/μg DNA/24 h; IGF-II, 0.25

± 0.5 nM/μg/24 h; mean ± = s.e.m., n = 4). Culture of islets with increasing concentrations of glucose between 2.7 mM and 16.7 mM did not alter the release of either IGF peptide.

The release of IGF BPs by isolated islets was investigated using ligand Western blot analysis. Four species of IGF BP were released by islets into conditioned medium of molecular size approximately 44-46 KDa, 34 KDa, 25 KDa and 19 KDa respectively (Figure 1). The largest species had the double band structure characteristic of IGF BP-3 while the 34 KDa form was identified by immuno-blot as IGF BP-2. The 25 KDa and 19 KDa forms correspond to the known molecular sizes of IGF BP-1 and BP-4 respectively. When islets were incubated with increasing concentrations of glucose the presence of IGF BP-2 and the 19KDa IGF BP increased in abundance between 0.7 mM and 8.2 mM glucose (Figure 1). The release of IGF BP-3 was not glucose-dependent.

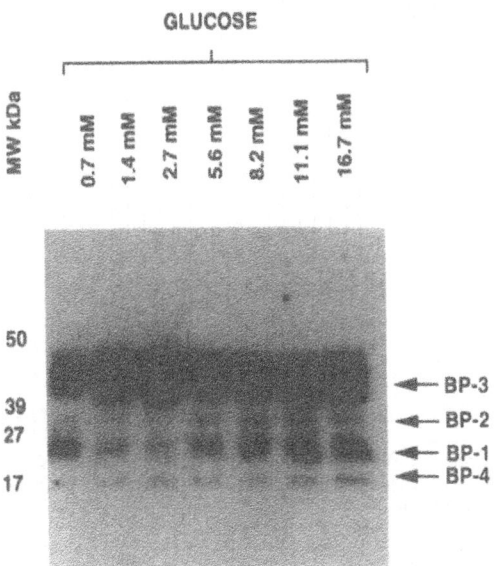

Figure 1. Ligand Western blot analysis of insulin-like growth factor binding proteins (IGF BPs) present in culture medium conditioned for 24h by isolated fetal rat islets of Langerhans. The ligand was [^{125}I] IGF-II. Molecular weight markers are shown on the left. Islets were incubated with increasing concentrations of glucose in the culture medium (0.7 - 16.7 mM). Four species of IGF BP were identified as IGF BP-1, -2, -3 and -4.

Islets were cultured for 24 h. in the presence of 8.7 mM glucose with or without increasing concentrations of exogenous IGF-I or -II and the DNA synthetic rate determined. Both IGF-I and IGF-II caused an approximate nine-fold increase in the incorporation of ^{3}H-thymidine into DNA. The ED_{50} of IGF-I was 1.8 nM and that of IGF-II was 8 nM. When the nuclear labelling index was estimated by autoradiography, 22% of nuclei contained ^{3}H-thymidine in control incubations, which increased to 27% in the presence of 6.7 nM IGF-I and 29% in the presence of 13.3 nM IGF-II. All cells demonstrating nuclear labelling were also shown to contain insulin by immunocytochemistry. The actions of exogenous hIGF BP-1 and bIGF BP-2 on DNA synthesis by isolated islets were also investigated. When added alone (2 nM IGF BP-1 or 1.5 nM IGF BP-2) neither IGF BP significantly altered DNA synthetic rate. However, in the presence of sub-effective (1 nM) concentrations of either IGF-I or IGF-II both IGF BPs greatly potentiated the mitogenic actions of the IGFs (Figure 2). IGF BP-2 was half-maximally effective in potentiating the actions of 1 nM IGF-I at a concentration of 1.5 nM.

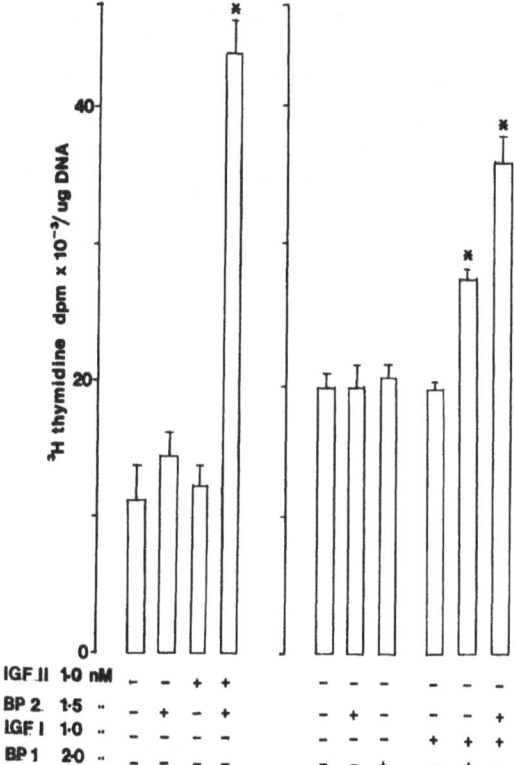

Figure 2. Incorporation of ^{3}H-thymidine into DNA by isolated fetal rat islets of Langerhans incubated with either sub-effective concentrations of insulin-like growth factor-I (IGF-I) or IGF-II alone, human IGF binding protein-1 (IGF BP-1) or bovine IGF BP-2 alone, or IGF-I or -II and IGF BPs in combination. Figures represent mean values ± s.e.m. for four replicate incubations. *p < 0.05 versus incubation with IGF-I or IGF-II alone. Two separate experiments are shown.

DISCUSSION

The results show that both IGF-I and -II are widely expressed in the developing rat pancreas, IGF-II being the predominant peptide during fetal and neonatal development while IGF-I becomes predominant around the time of weaning. At least two IGF BPs, IGF BP-1 and -2, are also expressed by the pancreas *in situ* with a maximal abundance of mRNA being present around the time of weaning. Isolated fetal rat islets of Langerhans contain and release both IGF-I and -II *in vitro* with IGF-II being the predominant form. Despite this release pattern IGF-I was substantially more active as a mitogen on isolated islets than was IGF-II. Immunocytochemistry showed that almost all the cells undergoing DNA synthesis *in vitro* and which respond to IGFs were β-cells. However, under these conditions the expression and release of IGF-I and -II by islets was not modulated by variations in glucose, although glucose was capable of acting as a mitogenic stimulus and an insulin secretogogue. However, islets contain and released at least four species of IGF BP of which one species was identified immunologically as IGF BP-2. The release of IGF BP-2 and another 19 KDa species by islets was positively regulated by glucose within the physiological range of glucose concentrations. In the isolated islet model exogenous IGF BP-1 or -2 potentiated the ability of IGF-I or -II to increase DNA synthetic rate. In several other cell systems IGF BPs have been shown to regulate the ability of IGFs to associate with cell membranes and to modulate IGF bioactivity, in both a stimulatory and an inhibitory manner.[24,29] It is therefore possible that IGF BP expression and release is the dynamic variable within the islet:IGF axis, and that a glucose-dependent change in IGF BP synthesis may modulate the actions of endogenous IGFs which are themselves released in a constitutive manner. The ability of glucose to modulate islet cell DNA synthesis may therefore be mediated, in part, by changes in the availability of IGF BPs. Since IGFs are expressed throughout the mesenchyme, exocrine tissue and islets of the developing pancreas, and are also potentially available from the circulation, complex endocrine/paracrine interactions are likely to occur. The ability of IGF BPs to modulate IGF mitogenic action is one way in which the target tissue can modulate locally the anabolic milieu.

SUMMARY

Growth of pancreatic β-cells is an essential feature of development in order to maintain insulin availability. While glucose has been shown to increase β-cell DNA synthetic rate in cultures of isolated islets of Langerhans, there is also evidence for a local control of β-cell growth involving insulin-like growth factors (IGFs). IGF I and II and their specific binding proteins (IGF BPs) are expressed within the developing rat pancreas, and released by isolated fetal rat islets of Langerhans. Glucose-induced β-cell growth is not mediated by IGF-I, since IGF release does not alter in response to changes in glucose availability. In contrast, IGF BP release is positively associated with glucose concentrations over the physiological range and is therefore a candidate. Exogenous hIGF BP1 or bIGF BP2 synergistically interacted with hIGF I or II to increase DNA synthesis within isolated fetal rat islets. These results suggest a role for IGF BPs in the regulation of β-cell growth. They may act independently or by modulation of IGF bioavailability during pancreatic development.

REFERENCES

1. D.J. Hill, D. De Sousa, Insulin is a mitogen for isolated epiphyseal growth plate chondrocytes from the fetal lamb, Endocrinology. 126:2661-70 (1990).
2. I. Swenne, U. Eriksson, Diabetes in pregnancy: Islet cell proliferation in fetal rat pancreas, Diabetologia. 23:525-28 (1982).
3. B. Portha, C. Levacher, L. Picon, G. Rosselin, Diabetogenic effect of streptozotocin in the rat during the perinatal period, Diabetes. 23:889-95 (1974).
4. M. De Gasparo, G.R. Milner, P.D. Norris, R.D.G. Milner, Effect of glucose and amino acids on fetal rat pancreatic growth and insulin secretion *in vitro*, J Endocrinology. 77:241-48 (1978).
5. L. Rosenberg, This Volume.
6. G.L. Pittenger, This Volume.
7. H. Okamoto, This Volume.
8. C. Newgard, This Volume.
9. N. Sarvetnick, This Volume.
10. V.K.M. Han, D.J. Hill, A.J. Strain, et al, Identification of somatomedin/insulin-like growth factor immunoreactive cells in the human fetus, Pediatr Res. 22:245-49 (1987).
11. D.J. Hill, D.R. Clemmons, S. Wilson, V.K.M. Han, A.J. Strain, R.D.G. Milner, Immunological distribution of one form of insulin-like growth factor (IGF) binding protein and IGF peptides in human fetal tissues, J Mol Endocrinology. 2:31-38 (1989).
12. D.J. Hill, unpublished observations.
13. D.J. Hill, A. Frazer, I. Swenne, K. Wirdnam, R.D.G. Milner, Somatomedin-C in the human foetal pancreas: Cellular localization and release during organ culture, Diabetes. 36:465-71 (1987).
14. V.K.M. Han, P.K. Lund, D.C. Lee, A.J. D'Ercole, Expression of somatomedin/ insulin-like growth factor in the human fetus: Identification, characterization and tissue distribution, J Clin Endocr Metab. 66:422-29 (1988).
15. I. Swenne, D.J. Hill, A.J. Strain, R.D.G. Milner, Growth hormone regulation of somatomedin-C/insulin-like growth factor I production and DNA replication in fetal rat islets in tissue culture, Diabetes. 36:288-94 (1987).
16. D.J. Hill, J. Hogg, J.F. Wang, D.R. Clemmons, Release of IGF binding proteins by fetal rat islets of Langerhans: Modulation of IGF-induced DNA synthesis. 2nd Int. IGF Symposium San Francisco, CA, 53 [Abstract], 1991.
17. R. Scharfmann, M. Corvol, P. Czernichow, Characterization of IGF I produced by fetal rat pancreatic cells, Diabetes. 38:686-90 (1989).
18. I. Swenne, C-H Heldin, D.J. Hill, C. Hellerstrom, Effects of platelet-derived growth factor and somatomedin-C/insulin-like growth factor I on the DNA replication of fetal rat islets of Langerhans in tissue culture, Endocrinology. 122:214-18 (1988).

19. A. Rabinovitch, C. Quigley, T. Russel, et al, Insulin and multiplication stimulating activity (an insulin-like growth factor) stimulate islet ß-cell replication in neonatal rat pancreatic monolayer cultures, Diabetes. 31:160-64 (1982).

20. T. Otonkoski, M. Knip, I. Wong, O. Simell, Effect of growth hormone and insulin-like growth factor on endocrine function of human fetal islet-like cell clusters during long-term culture, Diabetes. 37:1678-83 (1988).

21. C.F. Van Schravendijk, A. Foriers, J.L. Van Den Brande, D.G. Pipeleers, Evidence for the presence of type I insulin-like growth factor receptors on rat pancreatic A and B cells, Endocrinology. 121:1784-88 (1987).

22. J.J. Van Wyk, L.E. Underwood, A.J. D'Ercole, et al, Role of somatomedin in cellular proliferation. in: "Biology of Normal Human Growth," M. Ritzen, A. Aperia, K. Hall, A. Larsson, A. Zetterburg, and R. Zellerstrom, eds., Raven Press, New York. (1981).

23. A.K. Chatterjee, J. Sieradzki, H. Schatz, Epidermal growth factor stimulates (pro) insulin biosynthesis and ^{3}H-thymidine incorporation in isolated pancreaticrat islets, Horm Metab Res. 18:873-74 (1986).

24. R.G. Elgin, W.H. Busby, D.R. Clemmons, An insulin-like growth factor (IGF) binding protein enhances the biological response to IGF I, Proc Natl Acad Sci USA. 84:3254-58 (1987).

25. C. Hellerstrom, N.J. Lewis, H. Borg,, R. Johnson, N. Freinkel, Method for large-scale isolation of pancreatic islets by tissue culture of fetal rat pancreas, Diabetes. 31:160-64 (1979).

26. D.J. Hill, Relative abundance and molecular size of immunoreactive insulin-like growth factors I and II in human fetal tissues, Early Hum Dev. 21:49-58 (1990).

27. J.F. Wang, G.P. Becks, K.D. Buckingham, D.J. Hill, Characterization of insulin-like growth factor-binding proteins secreted by isolated sheep thyroid epithelial cells, J Endocrinology. 125:439-48 (1990).

28. D.J. Hill , C. Comacho-Hubner, P. Rashid, A.J. Strain, D.R. Clemmons, Insulin-like growth factor (IGF) binding protein release by human fetal fibroblasts: Dependency on cell density and IGF peptides, J Endocrinol. 122:87-98 (1989).

29. W.M. Burch, J. Correa, J.E. Shively, D.R. Powell, The 25-kilodalton insulin-like growth factor (IGF)-binding protein inhibits both basal and IGF-I-mediated growth of chick embryo pelvic cartilage in vitro, J Clin Endocrinol Metab. 70:173-80 (1990).

DISCUSSION

C. Newgard: I was just wondering whether all of these studies are on fetal islets?

D. Hill: Yes.

C. Newgard: Can you reproduce any of these nice effects that you are seeing on adult islets?

D. Hill: We've not really done these experiments with adult islets. We have worked with adult islets to show that they will release IGF-1 in culture although it's not as dramatic as we see with IGF-2 in the fetal system. The release of IGF-1 in those adult islets seems to be potentiated by growth in the same way as we've seen in late gestation in fetal islets. The effects of growth hormone on DNA synthesis could not be completely blocked with an anti-IGF-1 antibody in the adult. So I believe there is probably some direct effect of growth hormone in the adult system, it's not only mediated through the IGF system.

C. Newgard: Just a quick follow-up on that. You're isolating the fetal islets, and you talked about the necessity for hyperplasia to accompany the rapid burst in body mass, is that correct? And is it possible that when you isolate fetal islets there are some residual components of proliferation that allow you to see these effects which won't be there in the adult islets. To ask that another way; when you isolate fetal islets, do you see a couple rounds of cell division that then subside right after isolation, or how does that go?

D. Hill: Well, our period of studies reported are 48 hours to as short as an hour after a 5-day incubation. We haven't taken them out further than that. You can also see an awful lot of mitotic figures. So yes, I'd be very happy to believe that you are seeing the residual hyperplastic effect.

A. Vinik: David, we missed you this morning because what was shown by Jens is that the growth hormone had an effect on newborn rat islets which was independent of IGF-1. Would you concur?

J. Nielsen: Is it likely that growth hormone has a direct effect? In our model using fetal tissues, islet growth occurs with IGFs and their binding proteins. Have you done any experiments with more specific identification of the islets or the cells incorporating thymidine.

D. Hill: Well, we took the duct cells and studied them for nuclear labeling effects but I don't think we're looking at mitotic figures. I think we are looking at new cell development. There must be growth factors in there somewhere. What they are, whether they are matrix components, stabilizing the islets in some way, or whether it's the key growth factor that is active in very, very low amounts, I don't know.

A. Vinik:	Your experiments demonstrating release of IGF bring up the issue of whether or not, in the process of isolation, you isolate binding protein which directs the focus of the growth factor to the particular islet. Now is that what's presented or are there insufficient quantities of protein to generate the complex?
D. Hill:	If you look at the IGF-1 and 2 distribution in fetal islets then it's all there, a complex product of binding protein and IGFs. So I think that there is an excess of binding protein there.
A. Vinik:	If there is an excess of binding protein there, why then are you getting effects on growth when you administer IGFs with more binding protein?
D. Hill:	Because when you add more binding protein, you probably accomplish extraction since there is no endigenous binding protein to get the most out of the IGF-2 cells. If you add more IGF-1, you overcome the available binding protein then you see effects of IGF-1. So right, if you added excessive IGF binding protein, you get a potentiation of the effect of IGF.
A. Vinik:	You are suggesting, then, that the endogenous protein -if it is endogenous IGF-binding protein - is not actually binding in such a way to yield an optimum ratio of binding protein to IGF?
D. Hill:	Well, what we are assuming is that the binding protein is made endogenously and is already bringing out the endogenous IGF. What this experiment examines is the interaction between excess binding protein and available IGF.
A. Vinik:	How does the IGF added compare to the quantitiy of IGF that is actually released?
D. Hill:	Well, it is very difficult to estimate the actual amount released. When you look at release you look at small amounts in a large volume. There is simply too much error in doing these estimates.
A. Vinik:	What you need to get a biological response is a one to two nonamolar of exogenous IGF-1. So are we in the right ballpark?
D. Hill:	If you assume that some of the IGF is not going to be freely diffusible in the volume of buffer used *in vitro*, and that maybe it's going to be held close to the islets by the binding proteins, then I think our notion is physiologically valid.
A. Vinik:	It would be nice to see what would happen to mature adult cells treated with IGF's and their binding proteins.
C. Newgard:	You know what's interesting about that, though, is that high glucose tends to make the islet become phenotypically mature. In the sense that they become glucose responsive to high glucose - if I remember the original data - but do not become glucose responsive at low glucose levels. So there is a sort of a paradox here; there is still a replication response, or the cells are geared up for replication and yet they appear to be differentiated in the sense of glucose sensitivity.

THE PARTIAL ISOLATION AND CHARACTERIZATION OF ILOTROPIN, A NOVEL ISLET-SPECIFIC GROWTH FACTOR

Gary L. Pittenger, Ph.D.,[1] Aaron I. Vinik, M.D., Ph.D.,[1]
Lawrence Rosenberg, M.D., Ph.D.[2]

[1]Eastern Virginia Medical School
 Diabetes Institutes
 855 West Brambleton Ave.
 Norfolk, VA. 23510

[2]Lawrence Rosenberg, M.D., Ph.D.
 McGill University
 Montreal Hospital
 Montreal, Quebec

INTRODUCTION

A reduction of the β-cell mass in the pancreas is the critical clinical event in the development of insulin-dependent diabetes mellitus (IDDM), and a reduced islet mass, in combination with insulin resistance, is necessary for non-insulin dependent diabetes (NIDDM) to develop. The acute onset of disease is preceded by a period of progressive destruction of pancreatic islets without replacement, until the remaining mass is insufficient to respond to hyperglycemia. It would, therefore, be of interest to examine the regulation of islet cell growth, and the factors that prevent or promote replacement of the lost islets. A number of animal models of IDDM have been developed for investigation of these processes, with the aim of preventing diabetes by reversing the loss of islets through β-cell destruction.[1-3] It is evident that regeneration and maintenance of pancreatic endocrine tissue after the onset of islet destruction would have significant therapeutic impact on diabetes mellitus.

We have shown, in a series of studies, that cellophane wrapping the head of the pancreas in Syrian golden hamsters induces the growth, differentiation, and proliferation of new islet tissue. One major difference between our model and the others presented in this symposium is that, while effects on extant islets cannot be ruled out, islet growth and repopulation of the pancreas in the cellophane wrapped model is predominantly a result of the differentiation of endocrine tissue from duct epithelium. This difference is demonstrated by studies showing an increase in the number of small, new islets associated with duct epithelium,[4,5] the increased uptake of ^{3}H-thymidine by duct epithelium in response to wrapping,[6] and the reversal of steptozotocin-induced diabetes by cellophane wrapping the pancreas.[7,8] Therefore, we asked the question, "What is the nature of the stimulus which results in the growth of new islet tissue in the cellophane wrap model?"

Many modes of cell-to-cell interaction have been described for the growing family of known growth promoters. Signaling over distances in the body can be accomplished by endocrine (hormone) or exocrine (lumone) pathways. Local signaling can also be delivered via paracrine, autocrine and juxtacrine cellular interactions. Parabiotic experiments using the cellophane wrapping model have strongly suggested that the growth-promoting activity is exerted locally, from within the pancreas, rather than acting through systemic distribution,[9] although the parabiotic experiments do not preclude delivery of subthreshold amounts in a classical hormonal schema. This implies that both the cells of origin and the target cells are located in the pancreas. Thus, it is apparent from these results that if a growth factor is involved in regulating islet differentiation and proliferation, the factor acts in either a paracrine, autocrine or juxtacrine manner. This led us to hypothesize that there is a soluble polypeptide growth factor in regenerating pancreas. This factor is responsible for regulating the initiation of growth, proliferation, differentiation, and growth of new islets from duct epithelium in the cellophane wrap model of regeneration, and is likely to be capable, upon appropriate administration, of inducing the same type of growth as that described in response to wrapping the head of the pancreas in cellophane. It is this novel, pancreatic islet-specific factor that we call ilotropin.

PREPARATION OF CYTOSOL EXTRACT FROM WRAPPED PANCREAS - ILOTROPIN

Previous studies have shown that there is increased incorporation of ^{3}H-thymidine by duct epithelium in response to cellophane wrapping, with the incorporation peaking at about 2 weeks post-surgery.[6] Thus, it seems reasonable that there would be significant growth promoting activity at 10 days after the surgery. In order to test for the presence of ilotropin, a cytosol extract of regenerating hamster pancreas was prepared by excising wrapped hamster pancreata 10 days after surgery and homogenizing at 4°C in a salt buffer containing trypsin inhibitor. The homogenate was centrifuged at 140,000xg and the supernatant collected. To test for bioactivity, the extract was injected into 7-8 week old female Syrian golden hamsters twice daily for 2 days, and the pancreata excised for evaluation of induction of pancreatic growth. Injections of cytosol extract prepared from wrapped pancreata induced a significant increase in pancreatic weight and pancreatic DNA content when compared to saline injected controls (Table 1). Furthermore, there was a significant increase in islet number in hamsters injected with cytosol extract for 3 weeks compared to saline injected controls, similar to the response described previously[4,5] for the cellophane wrapped model. Thus, it appears that when a cytosol extract is prepared from regenerating pancreata in this fashion, it contains a factor that is capable of inducing pancreatic growth independent of cellophane-wrapping.

Table 1. The effects of pancreatic cytosol extract injections on pancreatic and islet growth in Syrian golden hamsters.

Group	Panc. Wt. g/100g Body Wt	DNA Content mg/100g Body Wt	Panc. Protein mg/100g Body Wt	# Islets/mm^2
Control	130±17	795 ± 159	21.2 ± 2.9	0.9 ± 0.5
Wrapped *	167±21	1052 ± 20	25.4 ± 2.7	1.8 ± 0.7

* Significantly different (p< 0.05)

CANDIDATES FOR ISLET GROWTH PROMOTER

The pancreas is known to both produce and respond to a number of soluble peptide growth factors, e.g., IGF-I, IGF-II, EGF.[10-15] In addition, several proteins have been shown to have enhanced expression under conditions that induce islet regeneration. Studies by Smith et al[16] demonstrated an enhanced expression of IGF-I in the 90% pancreatectomized rat. The *reg* gene was discovered due to enhanced expression in the rat after 90% pancreatectomy followed by nicotinamide treatment.[17,18] The apparent enhancement of growth factors in other models of islet regeneration suggested that ilotropin is likely to be markedly enhanced in wrapped pancreas compared to unwrapped. In order to test the possibility that the pancreatic growth was a result of the enhanced expression of a known growth factor, cytosol extract from both wrapped and control pancreata was tested by radioimmunoassay for a number of peptides and polypeptides. However, this preliminary testing for the active material in the cytosol extract revealed little new information. Table 2 shows a list of the known hormones and growth factors that were tested for, in both wrapped pancreas cytosol extract and in cytosol extract from untreated pancreata. These factors have been shown to have effects on the pancreas, and therefore have potential for promoting islet cell growth. In all cases the peptides tested were found in comparable amounts in both the wrapped and the control cytosol extract, suggesting that none of the factors tested was causing the islet growth seen in the cellophane-wrapped pancreas.

Table 2. Relative amounts of gut peptides and growth factors in pancreatic cytosol extract as determined by radioimmunoassay.

Peptide/Protein	Control	Wrapped
Insulin	+	+
Glucagon	+	+
PP	+	+
Glicentin	+	+
Bombesin	+	+
Somatostatin	-	-
CCK	-	-
EGF	-	-
Gastrin	-	-
VIP	-	-
Substance P	-	-
Motilin	-	-
IGF-I	-	-
IGF-II	-	-
IGF-Binding Prots.	?	?

This preliminary screening supported our hypothesis that the cytosol extract contained a growth factor, as yet unknown. Although other models of islet cell regeneration have indicated that genes such as *reg* and their protein products are significantly increased in regenerating pancreas, and therefore might be involved in promoting islet cell growth, probes for these genes and proteins have only recently been available. Dr. Rafaeloff describes her efforts to determine the roles of these factors in the cellophane wrap model of regeneration in another section of this text.

CHARACTERIZATION OF ILOTROPIN

We further hypothesized that ilotropin was a protein or polypeptide, and proceeded with efforts to both characterize and purify the factor. Our first approach was to test the ability of ilotropin to withstand denaturation. Aliquots of cytosol extract were exposed for 20 minutes to one of either heat (65°C), 0.4% perchloric acid, or 85% ethanol at 4°C and centrifuged for

20 minutes at 26,500xg. The supernatant of the acid-treated material was neutralized and, along with the supernatant from the heated aliquots and the reconstituted pellet from the ethanol-treated extract, were tested for activity using the hamster bioassay, described previously. Significant increases in pancreatic DNA content and pancreatic weight compared to saline injected controls were taken as indicators of trophic activity. As seen in Table 3, neither heat nor ethanol precipitation blocked significant increases in pancreatic DNA in response to ilotropin, while acidified extract, although inducing greater DNA content than control injections, did not significantly alter pancreatic DNA content. Similarly, none of these denaturing treatments, including acidification, was able to reverse the significant increase in pancreatic protein content, expressed as mg/100g body wt, in response to ilotropin. However, trypsinization of the cytosol extract did abolish the increase in pancreatic weight. Thus, it would appear that ilotropin is a soluble, relatively stable pancreatic protein, capable of inducing pancreatic changes within 2 days of application. Based on these results, partial purification for subsequent studies was accomplished by pre-treatment with heat, acid and ethanol precipitation.

Table 3. The effects of denaturing conditions on the trophic activity of ilotropin as measured in the hamster bioassay. († $p < 0.05$; * $p < 0.0005$; ** $p < 0.0025$)

Treatment Group	Pancreatic Weight mg/100gm Body Weight	Pancreatic DNA mg/100gm Body Wt.
Control	276±23	1.047±0.177
Crude Cytosol	333±35*	1.495±0.358*
Heat-Treated	329±24*	1.464±0.283*
Acid Treated	333±34*	1.119±0.438
Ethanol Precipitated	310±32**	1.212±0.252†
Trypsin-Treated	284±38	

Our next study for characterizing ilotropin was to examine the protein composition of the partially purified cytosol extracts using sodium dodecyl sulfate/polyacrylamide gel electrophoresis (SDS-PAGE), to look for proteins whose expression might be enhanced in the wrapped compared to the unwrapped pancreas. Aliquots from both wrapped and unwrapped pancreatic cytosol extracts were applied to SDS-PAGE[19] on a 12% gel, electroblotted onto Immobilon-P[20] and stained with Coomassie Blue. As seen in Figure 1, there are 2 proteins between 30-40KDa that are enriched in the wrapped cytosol extract compared to the control extract. This was surprising in light of the fact that most growth factors have molecular weights below 20,000. However, this was our first indication that we might in fact be dealing with enhanced expression of specific pancreatic proteins.

To further isolate ilotropin in a bioactive form, partially purified cytosol extract was applied to a 2.5x75 cm Superose-12® FPLC column and eluted at pH 7.0 with an elution buffer of 50mM imidazole, 5mM dithiothreitol, 200mM KCl, and 5% glycerol (w/v). The absorbance at 280nm of the eluate was constantly monitored, and the protein content of each of the 2 ml fractions collected was assayed. The 1 ml fractions were pooled as indicated (Figure 2) to test for trophic activity. Five peaks could be distinguished in the elution profile of cytosol extract, with bioactivity detected in the pooled fractions representing the third and fourth peaks, as indicated in Figure 2. These fractions corresponded to a molecular weight range from 66,000-24,000. Because the bioactivity was split between the two peaks, we

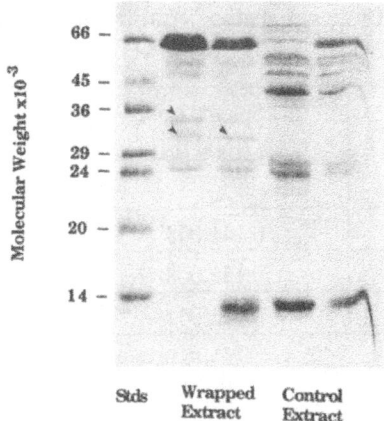

Figure 1. Wrapped and control pancreatic cytosol extract was separated by SDS-PAGE, and transferred to Immobilon-P for Coomassie Blue staining. Arrows point to two proteins enriched in wrapped cytosol extract compared to control cytosol extract.

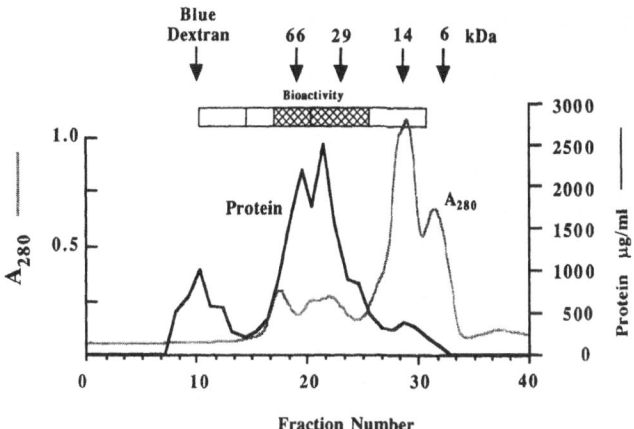

Figure 2. FPLC elution profile of cytosol extract from cellophane wrapped hamster pancreas as measured by absorbance at 280 nm and protein content of the collected fractions.

expect that the molecular weight of ilotropin will lie in the middle of this range, or approximately 44-29,000. This range includes the enhanced proteins seen in wrapped cytosol extract by SDS-PAGE separation.

Another common feature of many of the known growth factors is the presence of carbohydrate attachments, commonly sialic acid or mannose. For example, fibroblast growth factor was first identified as heparin-binding growth factor because of its avid binding to heparin affinity columns. To establish whether ilotropin might also be sialated, we passed cytosol extract over a heparin-agarose affinity column, and tested the heparin-bound and heparin-unbound fractions for activity in the hamster bioassay. As seen in Table 4, the material which remains unbound to the heparin-agarose matrix is able to stimulate increases in pancreatic weight (although not significant) and DNA content ($p < 0.05$), suggesting that ilotropin is not sialated, further ruling out a number of known growth factors as potential regulators of islet production induced by cellophane wrapping.

Table 4. A comparison of the trophic activity of cytosol extract components which bind to heparin and components which do not bind to heparin with saline injections in the hamster bioassay.

Test Group	Splenic Lobe Wt. g/100g Body Wt.	DNA Content mg/100g Body Wt.
Saline	0.14±.008	2.08±0.14
Lectin Bound	0.15±.008	
Lectin Unbound	0.17±.007	2.86±0.17

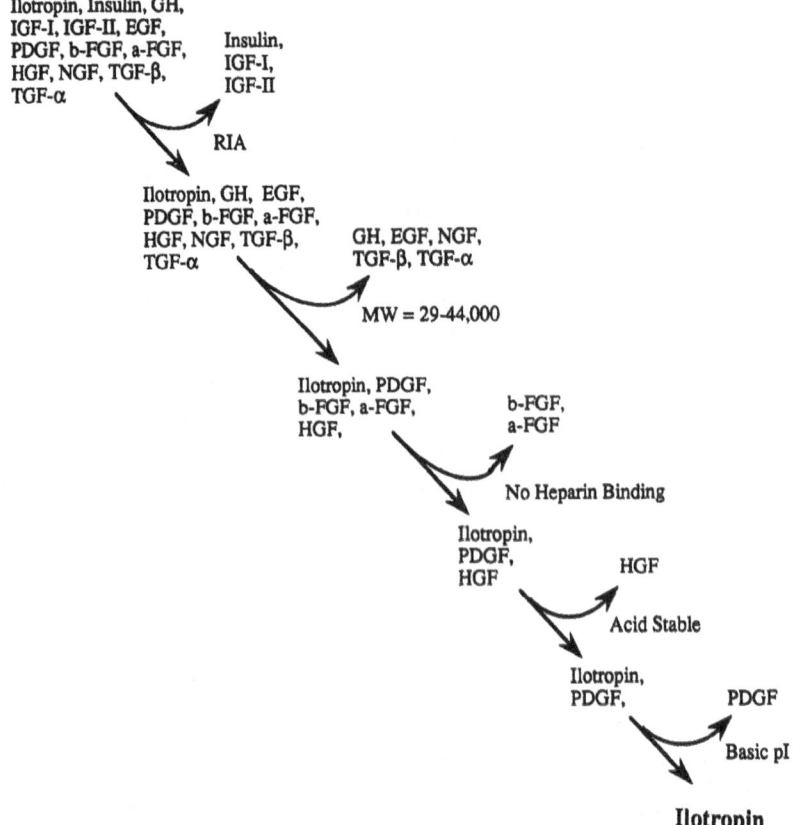

Figure 3. Flow chart showing the peptides and growth factors with potential for exerting islet promoting activity in the cytosol extract, and the elimination of the entire pool according to the characteristics for ilotropin described in these studies.

SUMMARY

In this series of studies, we have presented evidence for a novel, pancreatic islet-specific growth factor, which we call ilotropin. Ilotropin is acid stable, heat stable, ethanol-precipitable, and sensitive to trypsin digestion. It appears to have a molecular weight between 29 - 44,000, and preliminary data not presented here suggests that it has a relatively basic pI. Unlike many other growth factors, ilotropin does not bind to heparin.

Ilotropin is distinguishable from most of the known growth factors on the basis of at least one of the characteristics established in these studies. The apparent molecular weight of 29 - 44,000 eliminates all but the larger growth factors such as PDGF and hepatic growth factor. The fact that ilotropin is acid stable rules out identity with hepatic growth factor, and its lack of binding to heparin and apparent basic pI rules out identity with PDGF. Thus, the combination of characteristics described in these studies eliminates most of the known growth factors as candidates for the role of ilotropin. Certain growth factor precursor molecules (e.g. TGF-a) and several interleukins and cytokines (e.g. pro-IL-1 and melanocyte growth factor) also fall into this molecular weight range. Whether these proteins might be related to ilotropin or play a role in its biological activity remains to be determined.

Current studies of ilotropin include further purification to homogeneity, determination of the peptide sequence of ilotropin, and development of an *in vitro* bioassay using trophic responses of primary cultures of pancreatic duct cells as an indicator of ilotropin activity. With purified material we ought to be able to identify the cells of origin and the target cells for the action of ilotropin, and establish assays to determine the relationship to failure of β-cell regeneration that accompanies diabetes. Ultimately we hope that ilotropin may lead to new ways of approaching aspects of the problems presented in pancreatic β-cell failure.

REFERENCES

1. H. Okamoto, The role of poly(ADP-ribose) synthetase in the development of insulin-dependent diabetes and islet β-cell regeneration, Biomed Biochim Acta. 44:15-20 (1985).
2. J.S. Brockenbrough, G.C. Weir, and S. Bonner-Weir, Discordance of exocrine and endocrine growth after 90% pancreatectomy in rats, Diabetes. 37:232-36 (1988).
3. C. Miyaura, L. Chen, M. Appel, T. Alam, L. Inman, S.D. Hughes, J.L. Milburn, R.H. Unger, and C.B. Newgard, Expression of reg/PSP, a pancreatic exocrine gene: relationship to changes in islet beta-cell mass, Mol Endocrinol. 5:226-34 (1991).
4. L. Rosenberg, R.A. Brown, and W.P. Duguid, Induction of experimental nesidioblastosis - a model to study islet differentiation and function, Surg Forum. 33:227-30 (1982).
5. L. Rosenberg, R.A. Brown, and W.P. Duguid, A new approach to the induction of duct epithelial hyperplasia and nesidioblastosis by cellophane wrapping of the hamster pancreas, J Surg Res. 35:63-72 (1983a).
6. L. Rosenberg, W.P. Duguid, and A.I. Vinik, The effect of cellophane wrapping of the pancreas in the Syrian golden hamster: autoradiographic observations, Pancreas. 4:31-37 (1989).
7. L. Rosenberg, W.P. Duguid, and R.A. Brown, Effect of experimental nesidioblastosis on streptozotocin-induced diabetes, Surg Forum. 34:48-51 (1983b).
8. L. Rosenberg, W.P. Duguid, R.A. Brown, and A.I. Vinik, Induction of nesidioblastosis will reverse diabetes in Syrian golden hamsters, Diabetes. 37:334-41 (1988).
9. L. Rosenberg and A.I. Vinik, Paracrine/autocrine regulation of pancreatic islet cell proliferation and differentiation in the hamster. Studies using parabiosis, J Clin Invest. (submitted).
10. A. Rabinovitch, C. Quigley, T. Russell, Y. Patel, and D.H. Mintz, Insulin and multiplication stimulating activity (an insulin-like growth factor) stimulate islet β-cell replication in neonatal rat pancreatic monolayer cultures, Diabetes. 32:307-12 (1983).
11. I. Swenne, D.J. Hill, A.J. Strain, and R.D. Milner, Growth hormone regulation of somatomedin C/insulin-like growth factor I production and DNA replication in fetal rat islets in tissue culture, Diabetes. 36:288-94 (1987).
12. I. Swenne, C.H. Heldin, D.J. Hill, and C. Hellerstrom, Effects of platelet-derived growth factor and somatomedin-C/insulin-like growth factor I on the deoxyribonucleic acid replication of fetal rat islets of Langerhans in tissue culture, Endocrinology. 122:214-18 (1988).
13. T. Otonkoski, M. Knip, I. Wong, and O. Simell, Effects of growth hormone and insulin-like growth factor I on endocrine function of human fetal islet-like cell clusters during long-term tissue culture, Diabetes. 37:1678-83 (1988).
14. J.M. Bryson, B.E. Tuch, and R.C. Baxter, Production of insulin-like growth factor-II by human fetal pancreas in culture, J Endocrinol. 121:367-73 (1989).
15. P.J. Miettinen, Perheentupa J., Otonkoski T., Lahteenmaki A., Panula P. EGF- and TGF-alpha-like peptides in human fetal gut, Pediatr Res. 26:25-30 (1989).

16. F. Smith, K. Rosen, L. Villa-Kamoroff, G.C. Weir, S. Bonner-Weir, Enhanced IGF I gene expression in regenerating rat pancreas is localized to capillaries and proliferating ductules, Proc Natl Acad Sci USA. 88:6152-56 (1991).

17. K. Terazono, H. Yamamoto, S. Takasawa, K. Shiga, Y. Yonemura, Y. Tochino, and H. Okamoto, A novel gene activated in regenerating islets, J Biol Chem. 263:2111-17 (1988).

18. K. Terazono, Y. Uchiyama, M. Ide, T. Watanabe, H. Yonekura, H. Yamamoto, and H. Okamoto, Expression of *reg* protein in rat regenerating islets and its co-localization with insulin in the Beta cell secretory granules, Diabetologia. 33:422-24 (1990).

19. Laemmli U.K. Cleavage of structural proteins during the assembly of the head of bacteriophage T4, Nature. 227:680-685 (1970).

20. H. Towbin, T. Staehelin, and J. Gopdon, Electrophoretic transfer of proteins from polyacrylamide gels to nitrocellulose sheets: procedure and some applications, Proc Natl Acad Sci USA. 76:4350-54 (1979).

DISCUSSION

C. Newgard: How pure is the material at this point? If you ran it on a gel, what would it look like?

G. Pittenger: There are still a number of proteins. I didn't show any of the gels that we have, but there are quite a number of them. Our best bet are two dimensional gels. Apparently, again using a subtraction technique where we compare "wrapped" to control. We do have it down, probably, to five, maybe, ten spots, something that we can pursue.

C. Newgard: Do you see an increase in specific activity as you purify? In other words, does the same amount of protein have a greater effect with the pure material as compared to the crude extract?

G. Pittenger: So far we have not seen that effect, but I don't know that we've gotten sufficient purity for a biological assay. What we do is to take an equivalent amount of purified material that we started with and that is what we inject for the bioassay.

D. Hill: May I suggest another stab in the dark - I am suggesting a growth factor called the hepatocyte growth factor, published as a sequence in Nature a couple of weeks ago. It's the most potent growth factor ever found for isolated hepatocytes, and it works at very low picomolar concentrations. It's said to be expressed in the endocrine pancreas amongst other sites. We obtained some human islets a few months ago from a patient. There was a chance to put them through for our transplant program. But the donor was only 18 months old so we couldn't use them for the transplant synthesis program. So we did some biological studies on those islets, and these are purely anecdotal on one patient. One thing we did was to set up some 3H-TdR uptake experiments to get an idea of DNA synthesis response to hepatocyte growth factors. At 18 months these islets are still responsive to IGF-1 and 2. We've got about a three-fold increase in 3H-TdR uptake above those levels in controls. So what happens in response to the hepatocyte growth factor then? It turned out to be two orders of magnitude more potent than IGF-1. The only problem is that I think its molecular weight is about 36kD.

L. Rosenberg: Apparently, the trophic activity level of hepatocyte growth factor is heat labile and the material that Gary has described is heat stable.

A. Vinik: Nonetheless, one of the things we're going to do is to run the hepatocyte growth factor on the gels to compare to the extract to see if they co-exist or if they are similar in any way.

C. Newgard: You've done some size chromotography. Have you done a separation based on charge? Some of those growth factors like IGF are highly basic.

G. Pittenger: We are working on that right now. The two efforts that we have made at that are the two-dimensional gels and we've also done some preliminary work with ion exchange chromotography, and it appears that it's a fairly basic protein. One thing that we have had problems with is that our elution buffer on the HPLC interferes with any sort of ionic separation that we try to do. So we have to go back, do the ionic separation first, determine which peak has bioactivity and carry on from there.

EXPRESSION OF GROWTH FACTORS IN A PANCREATIC ISLET REGENERATION MODEL

Ronit Rafaeloff, Ph.D.,[1] Lawrence Rosenberg, M.D.,Ph.D.,[2] and Aaron I. Vinik[3]

[1]Eastern Virginia Medical School
The Diabetes Institutes
Departments of Physiology and Internal Medicine
Eastern Virginia Medical School
The Diabetes Institutes
Norfolk, VA

[2]Montreal General Hospital
McGill University
Departments of Surgery and Pathology
Montreal, Quebec

[3]Eastern Virginia Medical School
The Diabetes Institutes
Departments of Internal Medicine, Anatomy and Neurobiology
Norfolk, VA 23510

INTRODUCTION

As an approach to "curing" certain forms of diabetes several models for regeneration of pancreatic β-cells have been developed but the sequence of events and the stimuli for proliferation are still unknown. Furthermore, the various models have not established that the recreation of ontogeny is faithfully followed with development of a physiologic functioning β-cell. The developing pancreas appears as a protrusion from the dorsal surface of the embryonic gut.[1] At this time the endocrine α cells differentiate within the epithelial cell matrix. Later, the attachment of the pancreatic primordia to the gut narrows, forming the pancreatic duct and the first lobulations containing the differentiating exocrine tissue appear in the body of the gland. During this process the endocrine cells pinch off from the pancreatic duct and form the islets of Langerhans.

The different islet cell types appear sequentially during development *in vivo*. In the mouse for instance, cells containing glucagon (α-cells) appear on embryonic Day 14, insulin (β-cells) at embryonic Day 17, somatostatin (δ-cells) at embryonic Day 19 and pancreatic polypeptide (PP cells) at birth.[2-5] Little is known of the sequence in humans and other species.

After birth a new series of changes in specific gene expression occurs, such that the expression of the set of genes already activated in the embryonic pancreas is modulated, and several new genes are turned on. It seems reasonable to propose that coordinated growth is dependent on the specificity of growth factors for various target cells within the primordial pancreas or the duct equivalent followed by a series of changes in specific gene expression.

Several models to induce exocrine and endocrine pancreatic regeneration without tumor formation have been developed in the last few years:

1. The model developed by Bonner-Weir and colleagues demonstrates regeneration of both exocrine and endocrine tissue in rats that have been 90% pancreatectomized.[6] In this model *reg* gene expression is increased 24 - 72 hours after pancreatectomy and an increase in IGF-I mRNA in proliferating ductules and capillary endothelial cells is also observed.[7]

2. Okamoto and colleagues developed a model in which 90% pancreatectomized rats or mice are treated with either nicotinamide or aurothioglucose (poly ADP-ribose synthetase inhibitors) resulting in exocrine and endocrine cell regeneration and increased *reg* gene expression.[8,9]

3. A model of rapid β-cell proliferation following tumor resection in insulinoma-bearing NEDH rats has been studied by Newgard and colleagues who showed a large but transient induction in *reg* mRNA levels.[10]

4. Another model has been suggested by Sarvetnick et al[11] in which immunodestruction of β cells in transgenic mice expressing INF-γ is followed by a regenerative process which appears to be similar to the events that occur during embryonic islet cell development.

5. Partial obstruction of Golden Syrian hamster pancreatic duct by cellophane wrapping as a means of stimulating pancreatic islet growth has been developed by Rosenberg and Vinik.[12,13]

Previous studies done in this fifth model, show the following characteristics:

1. Cellophane wrapping of the hamster pancreas provides a trophic stimulus that leads to ductular cell proliferation and the development of new endocrine tissue in the pancreas of the adult hamster.[13]

2. New islet tissue is observed as early as 2 weeks after the wrapping procedure and it appears to arise from the ductular epithelium.[14]

3. Electron microscopic and immunocytochemical examination of the newly developed islets, identified cells containing insulin, glucagon and somatostatin.[14]

4. The newly developed β-cells are glucose sensitive and release a biologically active insulin.[15]

5. Incorporation of tritiated thymidine (^{3}H-TdR) by duct epithelial, ductular cells and islet cells is increased after wrapping of the pancreas.[14]

The mechanism by which partial obstruction in our model induces cell proliferation and differentiation is as yet unknown. However, using a parabiotic experimental design, these processes have been shown to be mediated by paracrine and/or autocrine mechanisms,[16] since the non-wrapped parabiont does not develop any pancreatic changes.

We therefore hypothesize, that cellophane wrapping of the pancreas in the Golden Syrian hamster model, induces growth promoting genes, embracing growth initiation, proliferation and differentiation genes in the ductal, ductular and islet tissues in an orchestrated, sequential manner, compatible with the evolution of functional islets from ductal elements.

Previous histological observations and ^{3}H-TdR incorporation studies suggest that the new islet tissue indeed arises from cells in the ductular epithelium through a possible recapitulation of endocrine tissue development.

The question as to which of the known growth factors participate in the proliferation and differentiation of ductal cells arises. In the Okamoto model of regeneration induction of *reg* gene appears to be one of the factors involved in this process although this has not been found uniformly by others working in this field. In studies presented here we investigated the expression of *reg* gene in control rat and hamster pancreas and in regenerating hamster pancreas to determine if *reg* was implicated in the hamster as well as in rats.

METHODS

Animals

8 week old female hamsters were selected. At this age they are fertile, considered to be adult animals and respond better to the induction of cell proliferation than do older animals.

Cellophane Wrapping

We used the method previously described.[13] Briefly, a midline laparotomy incision is made. With the aid of a stereo dissecting microscope, the distal common bile duct and head of the pancreas are exposed and a 3 mm-wide strip of sterile cellophane tape is wrapped around the head of the gland and tied loosely in position.

^{3}H-Thymidine Incorporation

^{3}H-thymidine incorporation (^{3}H-TdR) was determined by injecting 5μCi/g ^{3}H-TdR i.p. 1 hour prior to sacrifice. The pancreas was excised and fixed in Bouin's solution and the tissue processed for autoradiography. A cell was considered labeled if there were 5 or more silver granules overlying its nucleus. The ductular and islet labelling index (% of cells labeled) was calculated.

RNA Preparation

Total cellular RNA was isolated from hamster pancreas or liver using the Chamczynski and Sacchi guanidine isothiocyanate method.[17] Poly(A)$^+$ RNA was selected by passage over an oligo(dT) column.[18]

Analysis of mRNA

For Northern blots, heat denatured total or poly(A)$^+$ RNA was separated by electrophoresis in a 1.2% agarose, 0.6% formaldehyde/MOPS denaturing gel and transferred to nylon membrane and crosslinked by exposure to ultraviolet light.

Hybridizations were carried out in 30% formamide at 42°C (low stringency) and in 50% formamide at 55°C (high stringency) for 22 - 48 hours. Analysis of mRNA by in situ hybridization was performed on pancreas sections fixed in 4% paraformaldehyde and permeabilized with proteinase K, using a hybridization solution containing 50% formamide, 0.3M NaCl, 10mM Tris, 1mM EDTA, 2x Denhart's solution, 10% Dextran sulfate, 0.45 mg/ml sheared and denatured salmon testis DNA, 90 µg/ml yeast tRNA and 5×10^6 cpm of ^{35}S-labeled riboprobe. Slides were dipped in NTB-2 emulsion and stored in the dark at -20°C for 3 weeks.

RNA and DNA Probes

Riboprobes were generated from a human insulin cDNA of 510bp subcloned in pGEM4Z vector (provided by Dr. Graeme Bell) by linearizing the vector with NcoI or PstI and transcribing with SP_6 or T_7 for antisense and sense respectively, and from a rat *reg* cDNA of 726bp in pBluescript vector (provided by Dr. Hiroshi Okamoto) by linearizing the vector with PstI or KpnI and transcribing with T7 or T3 for antisense and sense respectively, in the presence of either [a^{32}P]CTP for Northern blots or [^{35}S]CTP for in situ hybridization. cDNA probes were labeled through the incorporation of [α^{32}P]dCTP by random priming.

RESULTS AND DISCUSSION

Trophic Effect of Cellophane Wrapping

The effect of cellophane wrapping on incorporation of ^{3}H-TdR into ductular epithelial cells was studied. Endocrine-like cells begin to form in association with the ductular-epithelium as early as 2 weeks after the stimulus of wrapping. The initial trophic effect of cellophane wrapping is on the ductular-epithelium (Figure 1) as shown by autoradiographic analysis following a single pulse of ^{3}H-TdR. The number of labeled cells per 2500 ductular epithelial cells was determined. The uptake of ^{3}H-TdR by ductular cells was maximal at approximately 2 weeks after wrapping, 4 weeks before the peak uptake of the label by islet cells.

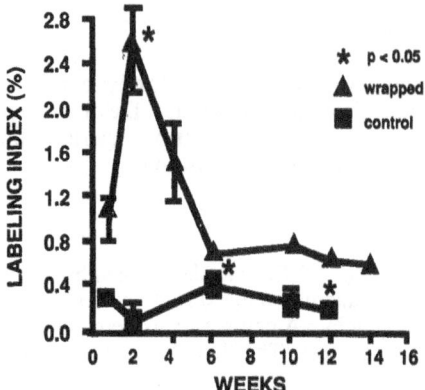

Figure 1. ^{3}H-TdR incorporation into DNA by ductular epithelial cells expressed as an index of percentage of cells labeled, in pancreas of Syrian golden hamster. (Δ) Labeling index for wrapped animals, ( ) control animals.

However, if the pancreata were examined 6 weeks after the pulse, most of the label was contained in differentiating islet cells, not ductular cells reaching maximal labeling between 8-10 weeks (Figure 2). Subsequent decline of incorporation to initial levels was observed after 14 weeks.

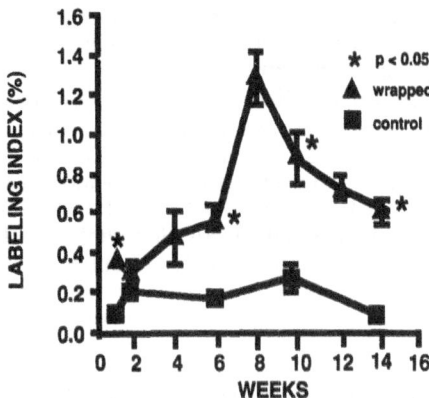

Figure 2. ^{3}H-TdR incorporation into islet cells expressed as an index of percentage of cells labeled, in pancreas of Syrian golden hamster. (Δ) Labeling index for wrapped animals, ( ) control animals.

The early proliferation of ductular cells demonstrated by maximal incorporation of ^{3}H-TdR at 2 weeks of wrapping, which preceeded the peak of islet cell labeling occuring at 8 to 10 weeks, together with the histological findings showing budding of neo-islet tissue from

136

ducts and staining of small clumps of endocrine cells among the exocrine parenchyma or in the duct epithelium, suggest that differentiating endocrine cells were derived from cells in the ductular epithelium. These findings could represent a reiteration of islet cell ontogeny.

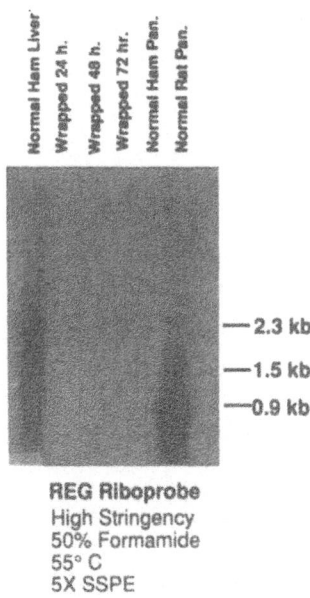

Figure 3. Northern blot analysis of *reg* gene expression in pancreatic tissue from normal rat and hamster and from cellophane wrapped hamster. The blots were hybridized with a rat *reg* riboprobe under either low or high stringency conditions. Each lane contains 30 μg total cellular RNA. 28S,18S and 0.9kb designate the migration positions of ribosomal RNAs and *reg* mRNA respectively.

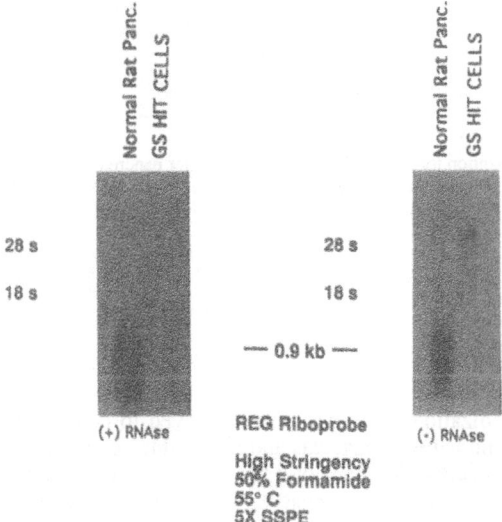

Figure 4. Northern blot analysis of *reg* gene expression in pancreatic tissue from normal rat and in HIT cells. Each lane contains 30 μg total cellular RNA. The blot was hybridized with a rat *reg* riboprobe at high stringency conditions and treated with 0.1 mg/ml RNAse A. 28S, 18S and 0.9kb designate the migration position of ribosomal RNAs and *reg* mRNA respectively.

137

REG and Insulin Gene Expression

Pancreatic tissue was excised from normal rat, normal hamster and from hamsters at various time points of cellophane wrapping and RNA was isolated as described in the "Methods" section. Northern blot hybridization experiments were performed on these samples using both low and high stringency conditions. Under both conditions there was an abundant 900 nucleotide transcript in normal rat pancreatic tissue which hybridized to the REG riboprobe but none was detected in either normal, regenerating hamster tissue (Figure 3), or hamster insulinoma (HIT cells) (Figure 4).

A. antisense

B. sense

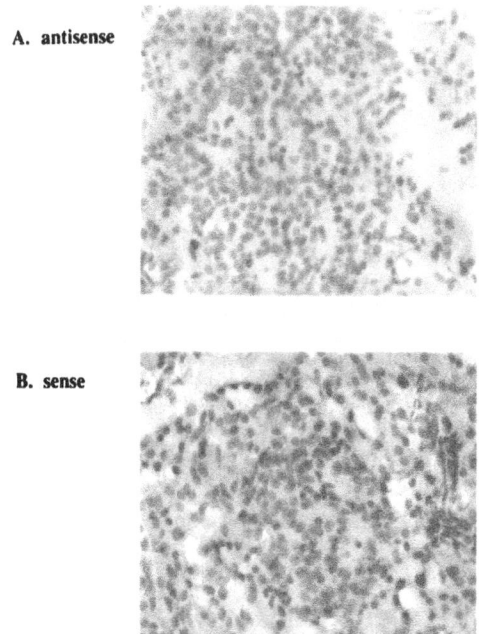

Figure 5. In Situ Hybridization for *reg* mRNA in control hamster pancreas ^{35}S-labeled single-stranded antisense (A) or sense (B) RNA transcribed from a 726bp *reg* cDNA were hybridized to sections of hamster pancreas and bright field micrographs were taken after autoradiography.

The in situ hybridization technique was employed to determine if the *reg* gene was detectable in control and hamster pancreas and if so, which cells expressed the gene. Figure 5 shows the brightfield autoradiographs of a section of control hamster pancreas where REG gene is obviously not visible. As a negative hybridization control we used a sense REG riboprobe.

Using an antisense insulin riboprobe, however, a strong hybridization was detected in the islets of Langerhans, whereas, the control, using the sense insulin riboprobe showed no hybridization (Figure 6).

138

A. antisense

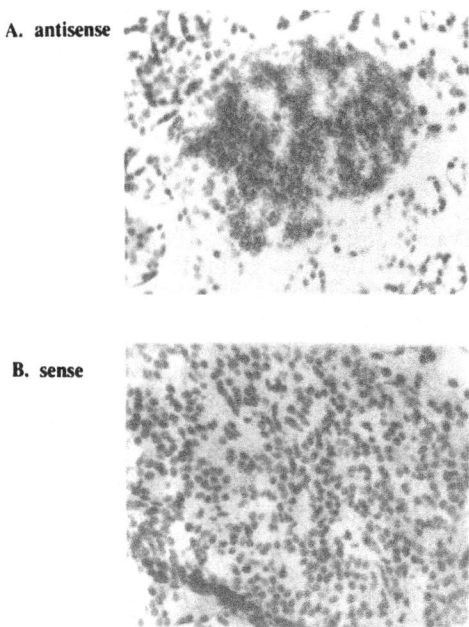

B. sense

Figure 6. In Situ Hybridization for insulin mRNA in control hamster pancreas ^{35}S-labeled single-stranded antisense (A) or sense (B) RNA transcribed from a 510bp insulin cDNA were hybridized to sections of hamster pancreas. Following autoradiography, bright field micrographs of the islet of Langerhans illustrate the expression of insulin mRNA.

A strong signal for insulin mRNA was also observed when using Northern blot hybridization analysis on poly A$^+$ RNA isolated from either control rat or hamster (Figure 7).

Figure 7. Northern blot analysis of insulin gene expression in pancreatic tissue from normal rat and hamster. The rat lane contains 5.6mg and the hamster lane 10µg of poly A$^+$ RNA. The blots were hybridized with a human insulin cDNA probe. 0.5kb designates the migration position of insulin mRNA .

SUMMARY

In this model of pancreatic regeneration, the initial trophic effect of cellophane wrapping is upon the ductular-epithelium, as shown by autoradiographic analysis following a single pulse of ^{3}H-TdR. The uptake of ^{3}H-TdR by ductular cells is maximal approximately 4 weeks before the peak uptake of the label by islet cells. Six weeks after the pulse, most of the label is contained in differentiating islet cells, not ductular cells. This phenomenom suggests that wrapping of the pancreas induces "progenitor" cells to differentiate along the line of endocrine cells.

The essentially negative observations on REG gene expression in the regenerating hamster pancreas indicate that the message for this gene is either not involved in the regeneration process or that it is sufficiently different from the rat gene (a rat control probe was used) that it precludes detection by our methdology. It might be necessary therefore, to generate a hamster REG specific probe in order to further study this issue.

In conclusion, the established model of cellophane wrapping of the pancreas provides a useful tool whereby the induced growth of β-cells can be observed. The sequence appears to be initial stimulation of ductal cells followed by islet differentiation. Of the candidate genes, it appears that *reg* does not participate in the process. We will however, examine other candidate genes to elucidate the mechanism whereby celophane wrapping induces growth of β-cells.

REFERENCES

1. R.L. Pictet and J.W. Rutter, Development of the embryonic endocrine pancreas, *in:* "Handbook of Physiology," D.F. Steiner and M. Frenkel, eds., Washington D.C., American Physiological Society (1972).
2. S. Bonner-Weir and L. Orci, New perspectives on the microvasculature of the islets of Langerhans in the rat, Diabetes. 31(100:883-89 (1982).
3. E. Samols, S. Bonner-Weir, and G.C. Weir, Intra-islet insulin-glucagon-somatostatin relationships, Clin Endocrinol Metab. 15(1):33-58 (1988).
4. G. Teitelman, T.H. Joh, and D.J. Reis, Linkage of the brain-skin-gut axis: islet cells originate from dopaminergic precursors, Peptides. 2(suppl. 2):157-68 (1981).
5. M. Yoshinari and S. Diakoku, Ontogenetic appearance of immunoreactive endocrine cells in rat pancreatic islets, Anat Embryol (Berl). 165(1):63-70 (1982).
6. S.J. Brockenbrough, G.C. Weir, and S. Bonner-Weir, Discordance of exocrine and endocrine growth after 90% pancreatectomy in rats, Diabetes. 37:232-36 (1988).
7. F.E. Smith, M.K. Rosen, L. Villa-Komaroff, G.C. Weir and S. Bonner-Weir, Enhanced insulin-like growth factor I gene expression in regenerating rat pancreas, Proc Natl Acad Sci USA. 88:6152-56 (1991).
8. K. Terazono, H. Yamamoto, S. Takasawa, K. Shiga, Y. Yonemura, Y. Tochino and H. Okamoto H, A novel gene activated in regenerating islets, J Biol Chem. 263:2111-14 (1988).
9. K. Terazono, Y. Uchiyama, M. Ide, T. Watanabe, H. Yonekura, H. Yamamoto and H. Okamoto, Expression of *reg* protein in rat regenerating islets and its colocalization with insulin in the β cell secretory granules, Diabetologia. 33:250-52 (1990a).
10. C. Miyaura, L. Chen, M. Appel, T. Alam, L. Inman, D.S. Hughes, L.J. Milburn, H.R. Unger, and C.B. Newgard, Expression of reg/PSP, a pancreatic exocrine gene: relationship to changes in islet β-cell mass, Mol Endocrinol. 5:226-34 (1991).
11. N. Sarvetnick, Islet cell destruction and regeneration in IFN-γ transgenic mice, J Cell Biochem. CB019:49 (Abstract) (1991).
12. L. Rosenberg, R.A. Brown, and W.P. Duguid, A new approach to the induction of duct epithelial hyperplasia and nesidioblastosis by cellophane wrapping of the hamster pancreas, J Surg Res. 35:63-72 (1983a).
13. L. Rosenberg and A.I. Vinik, Induction of endocrine cell differentiation: a new approach to management of diabetes, J Lab Clin Med. 114(1):75-83 (1989).
14. L. Rosenberg, W.P. Duguid, and A.I. Vinik, The effect of cellophane wrapping of the pancreas in the Syrian golden hamster: autoradiographic observations, Pancreas. 4:31-37 (1989).
15. L. Rosenberg, W.P. Duguid, R.A. Brown, and A.I. Vinik, Induction of islet cell proliferation will reverse diabetes in the Syrian golden hamster, Diabetes. 37:334-41 (1988).
16. L. Rosenberg and A.I. Vinik, Regulation of pancreatic islet growth and differentiation: Evidence for paracrine and/or autocrine growth factor(s), Clin Res. 38:271A, (1990).
17. P. Chomczynski and N. Sacchi, Single-step method of RNA isolation by acid guanidinium thiocyanate-phenol-chloroform extractions, Anal Biochem. 162(1):156-59 (1987).
18. H. Aviv and P. Leder, Purification of biologically active globin messenger RNA by chromatography on oligothymidylic acid cellulose, Proc Natl Acad Sci USA. 69(6):1408-12 (1972).

DISCUSSION

C. Newgard: Just a suggestion, have you thought about looking into Dr. Okamoto's homologous sequence of human and rat and finding identical regions? And using either PCR and oligos?

R. Rafaeloff: We've already got the oligos, that's exactly what I did. I looked at the homologous region, put it in the computer - used this beautiful program, called "Designer Primer" which helped me design these nice oligos. They are already in the freezer..

D. LeRoith: To follow up on that, with the oligos and PCR, so far as we see, there is a better chance for DNA contamination than we see on a Northern.

R. Rafaeloff: Yes, I mean we really tried to take one oligo from axon-2 and the other from axon-4 so that we wouldn't have any problems with genomic DNA contamination.

C. Newgard: It is bizarre that you haven't got hybridization with hamster RNA using the rat probe. It does not seem that it is due to RNA degradation, suggesting that hamster Reg may be different to that in the rat.

R. Rafaeloff: Yes, the RNA is clearly intact, as can be seen from the hybridization of insulin. We will have to wait to examine the PCR product to determine if these findings are due to a lack of sequence homology between Reg of the hamster and the rat.

ROLE OF p21^{ras} IN HORMONE SIGNALLING
AND CELL GROWTH/TRANSFORMATION

Peter F. Blackmore[1]

[1]Eastern Virginia Medical School
Department of Pharmacology
P.O. Box 1980
Norfolk, VA 23501

INTRODUCTION

This brief article will focus on the possible role of p21^{ras} in signal transduction. There is a plethora of conflicting information as to its function in cell signaling. Earlier studies suggested that p21^{ras} acted to couple certain membrane receptors to phospholipase C (PLC), which when activated, caused an elevation in inositol phosphates and a subsequent increase in intracellular free calcium ($[Ca^{2+}]_i$). However, more recent studies do not support this notion,[1] and suggest that the role of p21^{ras} maybe to alter transcription of transforming genes, thereby coupling hormone receptors to the activity of PLC. Evidence supporting this new concept will be presented.

PHOSPHOINOSITIDES IN CELL SIGNALLING

The actions of many hormones and growth factors are mediated by cell surface receptors, that when stimulated by agonists, elicit the hydrolysis of inositol containing phospholipids.[2,3] Two second messengers are produced following the phospholipase C cleavage of phosphatidyl inositol 4,5-bisphosphate. One is the water soluble *myo*inositol 1,4,5-P$_3$ which induces the release of Ca^{2+} from the endoplasmic reticulum. The binding site for *myo*inositol 1,4,5-P$_3$ is on the Ca^{2+} channel.[4] The release of Ca^{2+} from the endoplasmic reticulum causes an increase in $[Ca^{2+}]_i$. This increase in cytosolic Ca^{2+} alters the activity of many enzymes (e.g., phosphorylase kinase) that regulate many cellular functions. The other second messenger is the lipid, 1,2-diacylglycerol, which is an activator of protein kinase C.[5] This enzyme phosphorylates many proteins, some of which are enzymes whose activity are altered by phosphorylation.[5] It is clear from many studies that much of the 1,2-diacylglycerol produced following hormonal stimulation is derived from other phospholipids such as phosphatidyl choline, following phospholipase C activation.[6] The activation of various phospholipase C isozymes occurs *via* at least two different types of mechanisms. There are at least four types of phospholipase C (PLC) in mammalian tissues which are designated α, β, τ, and δ.[7] The identity of the α form of PLC, is however, in question. Each of the enzymes have similar catalytic activities to hydrolyze a variety of phospholipids. One form of PLC, designated PLC τ, has several *src* homology domains designated SH2 and SH3. These are highly conserved sequences found in many non-receptor tyrosine kinases such as *abl* and *src*. These SH2 domains interact with tyrosine phosphates found on several growth factor receptors such as those for epidermal growth factor and platelet derived growth factor. Following this interaction, the PLC τ enzyme becomes activated,[7] thereby causing the hydrolysis of phosphatidyl inositol 4,5-bisphosphate to *myo*inositol 1,4,5-P_3 which then elicits an increase in $[Ca^{2+}]_i$ by mobilizing Ca^{2+} from intracellular stores.

The non-receptor tyrosine kinase *src* is able to phosphorylate the epidermal growth factor receptor on tyrosines, therefore stimulating its ability to phosphorylate and activate PLC γ. This provides a link between *src* and phosphoinositide hydrolysis.[8]

Many extracellular signals activate PLC *via* a guanine nucleotide binding regulatory protein (G protein). There are several G proteins designated G_s, G_i, G_o, and G_q. Each G protein is a heterotrimer composed of an α, β, and τ subunit.[9] The β τ subunits, which are located in the plasma membrane, act to bind the α subunits when they are in the inactive state, i.e., when GDP is bound. The β τ subunits have also recently been shown to alter the activity of certain adenylyl cyclases.[10] The α subunit responsible for activity PLC β is a member of the G_q class.[11,12] Formerly the G protein proposed to be responsible for activating PLC was designated G_p. G proteins have also been shown to be involved in the hydrolysis of other phospholipids such as phosphatidyl choline *via* PLC to yield diacylglycerol as well as phospholipase D to form phosphatidic acid.[13] Also it was proposed that the low molecular weight *ras* oncogene product p21[ras] may act to couple certain receptors to PLC, since this protein binds and hydrolyzes GTP analogous to other conventional trimeric G proteins.[14]

ROLE OF P21[ras] IN SIGNAL TRANSDUCTION

The *ras* genes are members of a large multigene family that code for many proteins with highly conserved amino acid sequences. Three forms of *ras* (H, K, and N) are believed to regulate signal transduction associated with the growth control in mammalian cells. Certain point mutations in the *ras* genes result in the formation of altered gene products of 21 kDa molecular weight (p21[ras]) which are able to transform many cells *in vitro* (e.g., NIH 3T3 cells) to a malignant phenotype. Cells over-expressing normal p21[ras] can also lead to malignant transformation. The p21[ras] is located in the plasma membrane and is modified first by farnesylation of cysteine 186, followed by proteolytic cleavage of 3 C-terminal amino acids. Carboxymethylation of the newly exposed C-terminal cysteine then occurs. Palmitoylation of cysteines 181 and 184 may then follow. Palmitoylation of p21[ras] is a very dynamic process, and it has been proposed that acylation and deacylation may have implications for the role of p21[ras] in signal transduction[15]

The biochemical properties of p21[ras] proteins include the binding and hydrolysis of GTP. The GTPase activity of transforming mutant p21[ras] proteins are impaired. Also the GTPase activity of normal p21[ras] is activated 100 fold by the interaction with a 120 kDa protein called GAP (GTPase activating protein). Transforming p21[ras] (codon 12 and 61 mutants) on the other hand are not activated by GAP. The mechanism by which GAP stimulates GTPase activity is not clear.[16] A major unresolved question is, "does GAP protein control p21[ras] (upstream model) or does p21[ras] control GAP (down stream model)?"[17] The levels of GAP are much higher than the levels of p21[ras]. GAP contains two SH2 (*src* homology) domains similar to those found in PLC τ and phosphatidyl inositol 3-kinase, and thus can bind to certain growth hormone receptors such as the platelet-derived growth factor receptor *via* these SH2 domains. The role of this physical association of GAP to the receptor is presently not understood.[17,18]

ROLE OF P21[ras] AND P21[ras] GAP IN SIGNAL TRANSDUCTION

The evidence to support a role for p21[ras] in the coupling of hormone/growth factor receptor to the activation of PLC analogs to the heterotrimeric G proteins, is lacking despite some early "provocative" evidence.[1] There is, however, evidence that K^+ channel activity can be inhibited by a p21[ras]-GTP-GAP complex after activation by the G protein G_k. These

144

data suggest that p21^{ras}-GAP either directly inhibits the coupling of G$_k$ to the K$^+$ channel (upstream receptor) or inhibits the association of G$_{k\alpha}$ with β τ subunits.[19,20]

GAP can be phosphorylated on tyrosine in response to platelet derived growth factor (PDGF) or epidermal growth factor (EGF), and by the oncogene products v-*src* or v-*fps*.[20] This tyrosine phosphorylated GAP can bind to the PDGF receptor, also c-*raf*, PLC-τ and phosphatidylinositol 3 kinase have been shown to bind to the receptor. The binding of GAP to the PDGF receptor does not require the presence of p21^{ras}. How this PDGF receptor -GAP- phosphatidylinositol 3 kinase complex generates a proliferative signal is not clear. The current evidence suggests that the target for p21^{ras} is the tyrosine-phosphorylated form of GAP complexed to the PDGF receptor.

Another potential role for p21^{ras} is in the "formation, movement and fusion of intracellular vesicles".[18] Many low molecular weight GTP binding proteins, which are related to p21^{ras}, have been shown to be involved in these processes.[20] For example, the *rho* gene produce is involved in actin filament rearrangement.[21] From these and other studies a novel role for p21^{ras} has been suggested.[18] Support for this comes from the studies of Parries et al.,[22] in which p21^{ras} increased the expression of bradykinin receptors on Swiss 3T3 cells. This caused a potentiation of inositol phosphate production induced by the mitogen. In the same cells the response to PDGF was attenuated, without the loss of cell surface PDGF receptors. Thus it was proposed that p21^{ras}, after interaction with its effector, "could control assembly of a class of cell surface receptors at specific sites in the plasma membrane".[18] We have performed experiments in Balb/3T3 cells transformed with p21^{K-ras} and p21^{H-ras} which lend experimental support to the notions expressed above. These will be briefly discussed below.

H$_1$-HISTAMINE RECEPTOR SIGNALLING IN BALB/3T3 CELLS TRANSFORMED BY V-K-*RAS* AND V-H-*RAS* ONCOGENES

The ability of various Ca^{2+} mobilizing agonist (e.g., histamine, epinephrine, bombesin, thrombin, serotonin, epidermal growth factor, bradykinin, serum and ATP) to elevate [Ca^{2+}]$_i$ in K-*ras* and H-*ras* transformed Balb/3T3 cells were examined. In normal Balb/3T3 cells histamine did not increase [Ca^{2+}]$_i$; however, in K-Balb cells histamine produced a rapid increase in [Ca^{2+}]$_i$. Histamine did not elevate [Ca^{2+}]$_i$ in H-Balb cells. Other agonists such as serum, ATP and bradykinin produced similar increases in [Ca^{2+}]$_i$ in both Balb and K-Balb cells. The ability of histamine to elevate [Ca^{2+}]$_i$ was dose dependent (K$_D$ to elevate [Ca^{2+}]$_i$ and approx 50 μM) and was blocked by the H$_1$-antagonist pyrilamine. Histamine elevated [Ca^{2+}]$_i$ by promoting both influx of Ca^{2+} and internal mobilization of Ca^{2+}. Radioligand binding studies using [^{3}H] pyrilamine, showed the presence of H$_1$-receptors in both the K-Balb and H-Balb cells, but not in the untransformed cells. These results show that there is a complex regulation of H$_1$-histamine receptors by viral *ras* transformation. K-*ras* and H-*ras* transformation result in the expression of functional H$_1$-histamine receptors but the H$_1$-receptor expression and Ca^{2+} mobilization are uncoupled in v-H-*ras* transformed Balb/3T3 cells.[23]

Transformation of normal rat kidney cells (NRK) by v-K-*ras* does not result in the expression functional H$_1$-histamine receptors as it does in K-Balb cells. Thus v-K-*ras*-induced transformation appears to have cell-specific consequences. However, in these v-K-*ras* transformed NRK cells vasopressin (antidiuretic hormone) was unable to elevate [Ca^{2+}]$_i$ as it did in untransformed cells.[24] This effect was due to the loss of vasopressin receptors on the v-K-*ras* transformed NRK cells as measured by [^{3}H] vasopressin binding. The effect of other agonists, such as the P$_2$-purinergic stimulus ATP, were not modified by v-K-*ras* transformation, thus in NRK cells p21^{K-ras} specifically altered V$_1$-vasopressin expression.

CONCLUSION

The mechanism by which p21^{ras} leads to cell proliferations is still unclear. There is much evidence to show that p21^{ras} binds, through GAP, to certain growth factor receptors (e.g., PDGF receptor) and phosphatidylinositol 3 kinase, PLC τ and raf. There is also some experimental data to support the notion that p21^{ras} alters the level of receptor gene expression.[22-24] Other evidence to support this idea comes from studies showing that p21^{H-ras} activates transcription factor PEA1 and the polyoma virus enhancer.[25,26] Therefore, p21^{ras} may result in altered transcription of transformation-related genes and hence tumor formation and not act as a coupling protein between hormone receptors in the plasma membrane and the PLC enzyme.

REFERENCES

1. I.G. Macara, Oncogenes and cellular signal transduction, Physiological Revs 69:797-820 (1989).
2. M.J. Berridge and R.F. Irvine, Nature 345:142-52 (1985).
3. J.H. Exton and P.F. Blackmore, Calcium-mediated hormonal responses *in:* "Endocrinology", L.J. DeGroot (ed.), W.B. Saunders Co., pp. 58-74 (1989).
4. T. Furuichi, S. Yoshikawa, A. Miyawaki, K. Wada, N. Maeda, and K. Mikoshiba, Primary structure and functional expression of the inositol 1,4,5-triphophate-binding protein P$_{LLOO}$, Nature 342:32-8 (1989).
5. Y. Nishizuka, Studies and perspectives of protein kinase C, Science 233:305-12 (1986).
6. J.H. Exton, Signalling through phosphatidylcholine breakdown,J Biol Chem 265:1-4 (1990).
7. S.G. Rhee, Inositol phospholipid-specific phospholipase C: interaction of the γ_1 isoform with tyrosine kinase, Trends Biochem Sci 16::297-301 (1991).
8. W.J. Wasilenko, D.M. Payne, D.L. Fitzgerald, and M.J. Weber, Phosphorylation and activation of epidermal growth factor receptors in cells transformed by the *src* oncogene, Mol Cell Biol 11:309-21, 1991.
9. A.G. Gilman, G proteins: transducers of receptor-generated signals, Annu Rev Biochem 56:615-49 (1987).
10. W.T. Tang and A.G. Gilman, Type-specific regulation of adenylyl cyclase by G protein $\beta\gamma$ subunits, Science 254:1500-03 (1991).
11. M. Strathmann and M.I. Simon, G protein diversity: A distinct class of α subunits is present in vertebrates and invertebrates, Proc Natl Acad Sci USA 87:9113-17 (1990).
12. S.J. Taylor and J.H. Exton, Two alpha subunits of the G$_q$ class of G proteins stimulate phosphoinositide phospholipase c-b1 activity, FEBS Lett 286:214-6 (1991).
13. S.B. Bocckino, P.F. Blackmore, P.B. Wilson, and J.H. Exton, Phosphatidate accumulation in hormone-treated hepatocytes via a phospholipase D mechanism,J Biol Chem, 262:15309-15 (1987).
14. M.J. Berridge, The molecular basis of communication within the cell, Scientific American. 253:142-52 (1985).
15. R.J.A. Grand and D. Owen, The biochemistry of *ras* p^{21}, Biochem J 279:609-31 (1991).
16. C.J. Marshall, The *ras* oncogenes, J Cell Sci Suppl. 10:157-69 (1988).
17. A. Hall, *Ras* and GAP - Who's controlling whom?, Cell. 61:921-23 (1990).
18. L.C. Cantley, K.R. Auger, C. Carpenter, B. Duckworth, A. Graziani, Kapeller, and S. Soltoff, Oncogenes and signal transduction, Cell 64:281-302 (1991).
19. A. Yatani, K. Okabe, P. Polakis, R. Halenbeck, F. McCormick, and A.M. Brown, *Ras* p^{21} and GAP inhibit coupling of muscarinic receptors to atrial K$^+$ channels, Cell 61:709-76 (1990).
20. A. Hall, The cellular functions of small GTP-binding proteins,Science 249:635-40 (1990).
21. H.F. Paterson, A.J. Self, M.D. Garrett, I. Just, K. Aktories, and A. Hall, Microinjection of recombinant p^{21rho} induces rapid changes in cell morphology, J Cell Biol 111:1001-07 (1990).
22. G. Parries, R. Hoebel, and E. Racker, Opposing effects of a *ras* oncogene on growth factor stimulated phosphoinositide hydrolysis - Desansitisation to platelet-derived growth factor and enhanced sensitivity to bradykinin, Proc Natl Acad Sci USA 84:2648-52 (1987).
23. S.G. Oakes, P.F. Blackmore, and K.D. Somers, K-*ras* transformed BALB-^{3T3} cells express H1 receptors coupled to increases in intracellular {Ca^{2+}} not found in normal or H-ras transformed cells, FASEB J 4:A499 (1990).
24. S.G. Oakes, K.D. Somers, and P.F. Blackmore, Kirsten-*ras* transformed normal rat kidney (NRK) cells lose vasopressin receptors, FASEB J 4:A2987 (1991).
25. C. Wasylyk, J.C. Imler, J. Perez-Mutul and B. Wasylyk, The c-Ha-ras oncogene and a tumor promoter activates the polyoma virus enhancer, Cell 48:525-34 (1987).
26. C. Wasylyk, J.C. Imler, and B. Wasylyk, Transforming but not immortalizing oncogenes activate the transcription factor PEA-1,EMBO J 7:2475-83 (1988).

PHOSPHOINOSITIDES AND CELL GROWTH

William J. Wasilenko, Ph.D.[1]

[1]Eastern Virginia Medical School
Head and Neck Tumor Biology Program
Depts. Microbiology/Immunology & Otolaryngology
Head and Neck Surgery
P.O. Box 1980
Norfolk, VA 23501

INTRODUCTION

Phosphoinositides are a class of membrane phospholipids that serve as precursors to the important second messengers inositol$(1,4,5)P_3$ and diacylglycerol, which mediate the release of intracellular calcium and the activation of protein kinase C, respectively.[1,2] The key event in the production of these signals is the hydrolysis of phoshatidylinositol$(4,5)P_2$ by phospholipase C. This traditional pathway of signal transduction is utilized by activated receptors for a variety of diverse stimuli, including hormones, growth factors, neurotransmitters and chemotactic factors. Recently, several new pathways of phosphoinositide (PI) metabolism have been discovered in cells stimulated by growth factors or transformed by certain oncogene products.[1-3] These new pathways branch off the classical routes of PI hydrolysis and appear to be linked to poorly understood events in cellular regulation that are distinct from calcium release and C-kinase activation. In this discussion, several of these new aspects of PI metabolism relating to cell transformation will be illustrated, and a model for neoplastic transformation by the **src** tyrosine kinase oncogene, will be presented.

NOVEL ASPECTS OF PHOSPHOINOTIDES RELATED TO SRC ONCOGENE TRANSFORMATION.

Disruptions in signal transduction cascades are an important event in the transformation mechanism(s) of tumor oncogenes, as evidenced by recent discoveries that many oncogene products mimic receptor coupling proteins (ras), receptors (erb-b, fms) or growth factors (sis, int-2).[3,4] The **v-src** oncogene product, **p60-^{vsrc}**, is a 60 kD nonreceptor tyrosine protein kinase that is constitutively active and requires an association with cellular membranes for malignant transformation.[5] These properties allow **v-src** to alter a wide array of cellular parameters ranging from transport rates, cell morphology, gene expression, receptor expression and function; to name only a few. Recent structure-function analyses of **p60^{src}** and other activated tyrosine kinases indicate that many **src**-mediated events occur as a result of protein-protein interactions at SH domains within the amino-terminal portion of the **src** kinase.[3,6] SH (src homology) domains are highly conserved amino acid regions present in a variety of cellular proteins, such as growth factor receptors, coupling proteins, cytoskeletal components, etc., and they appear to facilitate interactions between proteins involved in the response of cells to many stimuli, including mitogens.[6] The presence of SH domains in the protooncogene product **c-src** argues for a role by the **src** kinase in cellular signal transduction events.

One of the earliest consequences of **src** activation is a stimulation of PI metabolism.[7,8] Initially, attention focused on the ability of **v-src** to elevate overall membrane PI turnover and PI(4,5)P$_2$ hydrolysis.[7,8] Recent findings now indicate these effects of **src** are complex and involve events occurring in newly discovered pathways of PI metabolism that branch off the traditional hydrolysis of PI by phospholipases.[3,9,10] (Figure 1) One of these pathways results in the expression of a novel family of phosphoinositides in the membranes of **src**-transformed cells that are phosphorylated at the D-3 position of the inositol ring.[11,12] These novel PI intermediates are distinct from the more abundant forms of PI, also present in **src**-transformed cells, which contain D-4 phosphorylations on the inositol ring.[1-3] Because the expression of these unusual D-3 phosphoinositides correlates with the activation of several tyrosine kinases, there is growing speculation these phospholipids may perform some important role as messengers.[3] However, none of the D-3 phospholipids appear to be hydrolyzed by phospholipase C.[1-3]

Correlated with the expression of novel D-3 phosphoinositide intermediates is a unique PI-3 kinase activity that associates with immune complexes of **v-src**, polyoma middle T/c-src complexes and several other activated tyrosine kinases including ros, v-abl and the receptors for PDGF, CSF.[2,3] Recent cDNA and amino acid analysis of purified PI-3 kinase reveal the presence of SH domains in a putative 85kD. subunit of this intriguing enzyme.[13] Furthermore, the enzyme appears to be tyrosine phosphorylated.[3,13] Thus, the activation of PI kinases and the expression of D-3 phosphoinositides are early events in the response of cells to several growth factors and tyrosine kinase oncogene products.

Additional complexities to PI signaling are also observed at the cytoplasmic level; namely, with the metabolism of inositol polyphosphate second messengers in activated cells.[1,2] In addition to the classic second messenger Ins(1,4,5)P$_3$ and its immediate breakdown products (InsP$_2$ and InsP$_1$), numerous other inositol phosphates accumulate in cells treated with a variety of agonists.[1,2] The additional inositol phosphates identified to date include cyclic inositol phosphates, Ins(1,3,4)P$_3$ and the higher order species of InsP$_4$, InsP$_5$ and InsP$_6$.[1,2] Of these, the inositol tetrakisphosphates (InsP$_4$) are particularly intriguing because several isomers of these molecules have been observed in stimulated cells; these include Ins(1,3,4,5)P$_4$, which derives from an Ins(1,4,5)P$_3$-3 kinase phosphorylation of Ins(1,4,5)P$_3$, Ins(1,3,4,6)P$_4$, and the enantiomeric pair D/L-Ins(1,4,5,6) P$_4$.[1,2] Although the function(s) of these diverse inositol phosphates in stimulated cells is unknown, their production does appear to result from a series of interconnected phosphorylation/dephosphorylation reactions, often with Ins(1,4,5)P$_3$ as a precursor. Thus, there is growing speculation that several of these inositol phosphates may have important roles in cellular physiology.

Although **src** and other activated tyrosine kinases cause significant disruptions to membrane PI, little is known about the downstream effects of tyrosine kinases on pathways of inositol polyphosphate utilization in the cytoplasm. To address this question, we are examining the effects of **src** tyrosine kinase expression on several parameters of inositol polyphosphate metabolism. Our model utilizes rodent fibroblasts (rat-1 cells) transfected with plasmids that allow for the expression of the transforming **v-src** kinase, or mutants thereof. To analyze the inositol polyphosphates, cells are labeled for 24 hrs. with ^{3}H-myo-inositol in growth medium. After the labeling, radioactive inositol polyphosphates are extracted from cells and analyzed by strong anion- exchange HPLC using gradients of NH$_4$H$_2$PO$_4$.[9]

In a typical experiment examining steady-state levels of selected key inositol phosphates in normal and **v-src**-transformed rat-1 cells, we find little effect of **v-src** on the cellular levels of Ins(1,4,5)P$_3$ and Ins(1,3,4)P$_3$; however, the **src**-transformed cells characteristically express marked elevations (6-7 fold) of an inositol tetrakisphosphate (InsP$_4$) (Table 1). Cells overexpressing the non-activated proto-oncogene, **c-src**, do not display elevations of InsP$_4$.

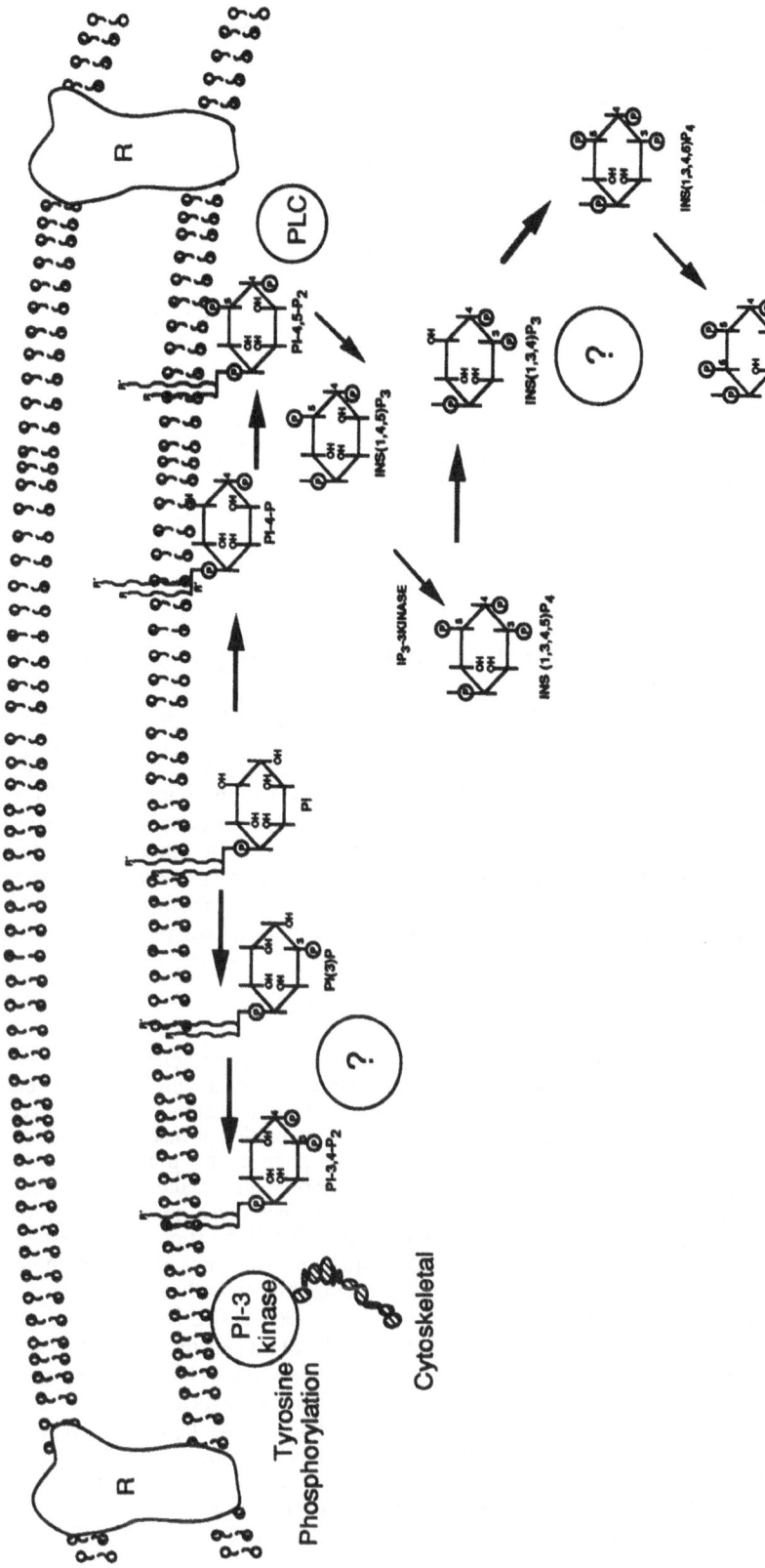

Figure 1. Novel aspects of phosphoinositide metabolism. The traditional pathway of phosphatidylinositol (PI) metabolism is shown on the right and results in the generation of the second messengers, inositol, (1,4,5)P3 and diacylglycerol (DAG). Branching pathways, affected by tyrosine kinases such as p60v-src, are designated by the circled question marks.

149

Table 1. Effects of V-SRC Oncogene Expression on the Steady State Amounts of Inositol Polyphosphates in Rat-1 Cells.

	Fold Increase Over Control		
Cell Type	Ins(1,4,5)P3	InsP4	Ins(1,3,4)P3
Normal Rat-1	1.0	1.0	1.0
Rat-1 c-src	1.2 ± 0.1	1.3 ± 0.7	1.1 ± 0.3
Rat-1 v-src	0.9 ± 0.2	**$6.2 \pm 1.9*$**	1.1 ± 0.3

Data represents the mean $\pm$ SEM from 5 experiments
Values were expressed as cpm/mg protein.

* $P < 0.05$ by one-tailed paired t-test

The elution characteristics of the elevated InsP4 in the **v-src** transformed cells are similar to those of the enantiomeric pair D/L Ins(1,4,5,6)P4.[9] Recent chemical characterization of this InsP4 isomer reveals it to be primarily D-Ins(1,4,5,6)P4.[10] The source of this unusual InsP4 is unknown, but recent findings suggest that cytosolic extracts from **v-src** transformed cells are capable of producing the novel InsP4 from Ins (1,3,4)P3.[10] Also associated with this unusual InsP4 profile is a marked elevation of apparent InsP3-3 kinase activity in **src**-transformed cells.[9] This enzyme is a calcium/calmodulin requiring enzyme that catalyzes the first step in the conversion of Ins(1,4,5)P3 to other higher order forms of inositol polyphosphates in cells, including InsP4.[1,2,9] Important areas for future study will be to establish the basis for InsP3-3 kinase activation in **src**-transformed cells, and the role this enzyme may play in the production of higher order inositol polyphosphates.

SUMMARY

The findings described above illustrate how the **src** kinase can influence several new pathways of inositol phosphate metabolism, both at the membrane level with the production of novel D-3 phosphoinositides and the activation of PI-3 kinase, and at the cytosolic level by altering the expression of certain inositol polyphosphates, in particular Ins(1,4,5,6)P4. At present, it is difficult to speculate on the role these phenomena play in cellular transformation by **src**, since the functions of D-3 phosphoinositides and most inositol polyphosphates are unclear. There is evidence, however, that these new pathways of phosphoinositide metabolism occur in response to other types of cellular stimulations besides **src** transformation. Novel D-3 phosphoinositides are expressed in a variety of non-neoplastic cells, including human platelets treated with thrombin, smooth muscle cells and stimulated neutrophils.[1,2] In addition, unusual InsP4 isomers such as D/L-Ins(1,4,5,6)P4 are found in chicken erythrocytes,[14] murine macrophages,[14] AR4-2J rat pancreatoma cells[15] and adrenal glomerulosa cells,[16] to name only a few. Recently, associations have been reported between PI-3 kinases and cytoskeletal elements in thrombin- stimulated platelets,[17] and between activated **ras** proteins in rat liver epithelial cells.[18] The latter discovery is particularly intriguing since GTP-binding proteins such as **ras** are known to influence cell shape and serve as downstream effector proteins in the siganl transduction pathways of numerous growth factor receptors. Thus, one function of novel phosphoinositides and their metabolites may lie at the level of cytoskeletal and cell shape regulation. Clearly, additional roles for phosphoinositides exist in cells besides their traditional use as precursors for the generation of Ins(1,4,5)P3 and diacylglycerol. Our future challenge will be to discern these roles and their relevance to neoplastic transformation and other cellular pathologies.

REFERENCES

1. M.J. Berridge and R.F. Irvine, Inositol phosphates and cell signalling, Nature. 341: 197-205 (1989).
2. V.S. Bansal and P.W. Majerus, Phosphatidylinositol-derived precursors and signals, Annu. Rev. Cell Biol. 6: 41-67 (1990).
3. L.C. Cantley, K.R. Auger, C. Carpenter, B. Duckworth, A. Graziani, R. Kapeller, and S. Soltoff, Oncogenes and signal transduction, Cell. 64:281-302 (1991).
4.. B.J. Drucker, H.J. Mamon, and T.M. Roberts, Oncogenes, growth factors and signal transduction, N Eng J Med. 321:1383-91 (1989).
5. J.T. Parsons and M.J. Weber, Genetics of src: structure and functional organization of a protein tyrosine kinase, Curr Top Microbiol Immunol. 147: 80-127 (1989).
6. C.A. Koch, D. Anderson, M.F. Moran, C. Ellis, and T. Pawson, SH2 and SH3 domains: Elements that control interactions of cytoplasmic signaling proteins, Science. 252: 668-74. (1991)
7. I.G. Macara, Oncogenes and cellular signal transduction, Physiol Rev. 69: 797-820. (1989)
8. Y. Sugimoto, M. Whitman, L.C. Cantley, and R.L. Erikson, Evidence that the Rous sarcoma virus transforming gene product phosphorylates phospatidylinositol and diacyglycerol, Proc Natl Acad Sci USA. 81:2117-21 (1984).
9. R.M. Johnson, W.J. Wasilenko, R.R. Mattingly, M.J. Weber, and J.C. Garrison, Fibroblasts transformed with v-src show enhanced formation of an inositol tetrakisphosphate, Science. 246: 121-24 (1989).
10. R.R. Mattingly, L.R. Stephens, R.F. Irvine, and J.C. Garrison, Effects of transformation with the v-src oncogene on inositol phosphate metabolism in rat-1 cells: d-myo-inositol 1,4,5,6-tetrakisphosphate is increased in v-src transformed fibroblasts and can be synthesized from d-myo-inositol 1,3,4-trisphosphate in cytosolic extracts, J Biol Chem. 266: 15144-53 (1991).
11. M. Whitman, D. Kaplan, T. Roberts, and L. Cantley, Evidence for two distinct phosphatidylinositol kinases in fibroblasts: implications for cellular transformation, Biochem J. 247: 165-74 (1987).
12. M. Whitman, C.P. Downes, T. Keeler, T. Keller, and L. Cantley, Type 1 phosphatidylinositol kinase makes a novel inositol phospholipid, phosphatidylinositol-3-phosphate, Nature. 332: 644-46 (1988).
13. M. Otsu, I. Hiles, I. Gout, M.J. Fry, F. Ruiz-Larrea, G. Panayotou, A. Thompson, R. Dhand, et. al, Characterization of two 85kD. proteins that associate with receptor tyrosine kinases, middle-T/pp60c-src complexes, and PI3-kinase, Cell. 65: 91-104 (1991).
14. L.R. Stephens, P.T. Hawkins, N. Carter, S.B. Chawala, A.J. Morris, et al, L-myo-inositol 1,4,5,6-tetrakisphosphate is present in both mammalian and avian cells, Biochem J. 249: 271-82 (1988).
15. F.S. Menniti, K.G. Oliver, K. Nogimori, J.F. Obie, S. Shears, and J.W. Putney Jr., Origins of myo-inositol tetrakisphosphates in agonist-stimulated rat pancreatoma cells. Stimulation by bombesin of myo-inositol 1,3,4,5,6-pentakisphosphate to myo-inositol 3,4,5,6-tetrakisphosphate, J Biol Chem. 265: 11167-76 (1990).
16. T. Balla, L. Hunyady, A.J. Baukal, and K.J. Catt, Structures and metabolism of inositol tetrakisphosphates and inositol pentakisphosphates in bovine adrenal glomerulosa cells, J Biol Chem. 264: 9386-90 (1989).
17. P. Grondin, M. Plantavid, C. Sultan, et.al, Interaction of p60c-src, phospholipase C, inositol-lipid and diacylglycerol with the cytoskeletons of thrombin-stimulated platelets, J Biol Chem. 266:15705-09 (1991).
18. A. Sjolander, K. Yamamoto, B.E. Huber, and E.G. Lapetina, Association of p21ras with phosphatidylinositol 3-kinase, J Biol Chem. 88:7908-12 (1991).

roles for phosphoinositides exist in cells besides their traditional role as precursor for the generation of Ins(1,4,5)P$_3$ and diacylglycerol. Our future studies will be to elucidate these roles and their relevance to neoplastic transformation and other cellular processes.

REFERENCES

THE PHYSIOLOGICAL STOP PATHWAY:
TARGET REGULATION OF AXONAL GROWTH

Francis J. Liuzzi, Ph.D.[1]

Eastern Virginia Medical School

Depts of Anatomy, Neurobiology Neurosurgery

Norfolk, VA 23501

INTRODUCTION

Axonal growth or regeneration is dependent upon a combination of intrinsic neuronal and extrinsic environmental factors. The interplay of these factors determines whether an axon grows, reaches an appropriate target and forms functional connections with that target. While many studies have focused on axonal growth and the factors necessary for that growth, relatively fewer studies, until recently, have addressed the question of how axons stop growing.

This chapter deals with that question and will discuss the physiological stop pathway. This concept was formulated by Liuzzi and Lasek[1] based upon their studies of dorsal root axonal regeneration and the failure of those axons to grow from the peripheral nervous system (PNS) environment of the dorsal root into the central nervous system (CNS) environment of the spinal cord.

MODELS FOR STUDY OF PHYSIOLOGIC STOP PATHWAYS

The lumbar dorsal root ganglia and the primary sensory neurons, which reside within those ganglia, provide ideal models for the study of peripheral nerve regeneration[2] as well as CNS regeneration. The dorsal root ganglion neurons are pseudo-unipolar neurons having peripheral axons extending out to either, skin, muscles, or joints and central axons extending into the spinal cord where they have extensive, stereotyped projections.

PHYSICAL BARRIERS TO NEURONAL GROWTH

After axonal injury, the dorsal root ganglion neurons undergo a number of changes. Peripheral axotomy is followed by morphological changes, called chromatolysis, or the axon reaction, which includes a dissolution of the basophilic Nissl substance, the rough endoplasmic reticulum of the neuron, movement of the nucleus to an eccentric position within the soma and enlargement of the nucleolus. These morphological changes are indicative of changes in gene expression and consequently, the synthetic profile of the cell. Transmitter synthesis as well as the synthesis of transmitter-related enzymes declines,[3,4] while the synthesis of proteins necessary for axonal extension and growth-cone motility increases. Moreover, the synthesis of the neurofilament triplet proteins, believed essential for the maintenance of neuronal size and axonal diameter,[5] declines.[6-9] These changes in the synthetic profile of the neuron characterize a reparative response of the cell to axotomy and signal the commencement of a growth phase.

Central axotomy resulting from dorsal root injury has a more subtle effect. There are no clearly evident morphological changes in the neurons, i.e., there is no observable

Pancreatic Islet Cell Regeneration and Growth, Edited by A.I. Vinik
Plenum Press, New York, 1992

chromatolysis or axon reaction. Yet, there are biochemical changes in the neurons that are less profound, but similar to those observed following peripheral axotomy.[9]

Just as the peripheral axons of the dorsal root ganglion neurons grow robustly in their peripheral nerve environment, the central, dorsal root axons, grow well within the peripheral nerve environment of the root. Yet, when the axons reach the dorsal root transitional zone, a PNS-CNS interface, the majority of them stop.[1] At this transitional zone, there is a dramatic change in the cellular environment encountered by the growing axon tips. Within the root, the axonal growth cones encounter the basal laminar tubes of the endoneurium made up of laminin and fibronectin, potent substrates for axonal growth.[10] Moreover, these tubes or bands of Büngner contain Schwann cells, which have been shown to up-regulate their synthesis of nerve growth factor following peripheral nerve injury.[11] Both of these conditions are favorable to stimulation of growth.

The CNS-side of the transitional zone, by contrast, has no basal laminar tubes. Moreover, astrocytes in the region react to the dorsal root injury by forming a characteristic glial scar.[12] This glial scar, composed of astrocytic cell bodies and tightly interwoven, hypertrophic astrocytic processes, have long been considered a physical barrier to axonal growth. However, studies by Liuzzi and colleagues[1,13,14] suggest that the transitional zone astrocytes are not acting as a mere physical barrier to axonal growth, but may exert a regulatory influence on that growth.

To address this question, Liuzzi and Lasek[1] used a very simple approach. If astrocytes of the transitional zone were acting as a mere physical barrier, the ultrastructural morphology of axonal endings in the region should resemble that of axons stopped at a physical barrier formed by tightly ligating a peripheral nerve or dorsal root. Studies were thus conducted in which the effects of a physical barrier were compared with that of transition zone astrocytes.

NON-PHYSICAL MECHANISMS FOR REGULATING NEURONAL STOP PATHWAYS

The ends of physically blocked axons were shown to swell immensely with membranous organelles, tubulovesicular profiles and neurofilaments. These swollen axon endings reached tremendous proportions and were measured at nearly 15µm in diameter.[1,15] However, when regenerating dorsal root axons reached the dorsal root transitional zone and formed axo-glial endings among the astrocytic processes of the region, their morphologies were quite different from those of the physically blocked axons. Axo-glial endings were small, having diameters similar to those of the normal dorsal root axonal presynaptic terminals. Moreover, the axo-glial endings were not characterized by accumulations of membranous organelles, but rather contained a small number of mitochondria and vesicles. In addition, like normal presynaptic terminals, axo-glial endings were devoid of neurofilaments.[1,13]

These simple, yet powerful, morphological observations indicate that the astrocytes of the dorsal root transitional zone, and the glial scar they form, are not merely a physical barrier to axonal growth. Rather, it appears that these cells activate an intrinsic stop pathway within the axonal growth cone. This physiological stop pathway is present in all axons and is normally activated when an axon reaches an appropriate target cell.

One part of the physiological stop pathway involves the breakdown and removal of neurofilaments, which are continually arriving by anterograde axonal transport at the axonal endings. Roots[16] showed that the breakdown and removal of neurofilaments from normal presynaptic terminals was protease-dependent. Similarly, Liuzzi[13] showed that the breakdown and removal of neurofilaments from axo-glial endings in the dorsal root transitional zone is blocked by intrathecal infusion of the protease inhibitor, leupeptin. Thus the same mechanisms at work in normal presynaptic terminals are at work in axo-glial endings.

Events at the ends of axons affect events back at the neuronal cell body where essentially all protein synthesis occurs. Activation of the physiological stop pathway, should then be expected to have profound effects on neuronal gene expression. And, this is the case. For example, there is substantial evidence that neurofilament gene expression and protein synthesis is regulated by axon-target interactions which activate the pathway.[7,9] Thus, there is an important negative feedback determined by axonal interaction with the target tissue. The nature of this pathway remains to be determined. There is, however, further evidence to suggest that both neurofilament gene expression and axonal growth are affected.

MOLECULAR MECHANISMS OF THE STOP FUNCTION

Hoffman and his colleagues[5-7] have demonstrated a relationship between neurofilament gene expression and axon diameter. After axotomy, neurofilament mRNA levels decline[4,7] as does neurofilament protein synthesis and transport.[6,8,9,14] Axon diameters consequently decrease.[5] When peripheral axons reach appropriate targets, neurofilament mRNA levels[4,7] as well as neurofilament protein synthesis and transport return to normal[6,9] and axon diameters increase. Similarly, when regenerating dorsal root axons reach the transitional zone, neurofilament mRNA[4] and protein synthesis[9,14] return to normal levels and axon diameter decreases.

When peripheral axons are stopped from reaching their targets, neurofilament protein synthesis stays depressed.[6,7] Similarly, when dorsal root axons are prevented from reaching the dorsal root transitional zone, neurofilament synthesis remains at post-axotomy levels.[14,17] These observations, coupled with the previous morphological observations[1] and the protease inhibition data[14] support the hypothesis that astrocytes of the dorsal root transitional zone exploit a normal pathway which is extant in axons and is normally activated when a growth cone reaches an appropriate target.

POSSIBLE MECHANISMS FOR ACTIVATION OF THE STOP PATHWAY

But what are the interactions between growth cone and target that activate the pathway? Membrane-membrane interactions are sure to be important and are likely to result in a cessation of growth cone filopodial extension. In peripheral nerve regeneration, growth cones interact by specific receptors with substrates of laminin and fibronectin.[18,19] Neither laminin[20] nor fibronectin [21] are detectable on the CNS side of the dorsal root transitional zone. Additionally, normal target tissues and CNS glia may use inhibitory surface molecules to regulate axonal growth. One such molecule may be chondroitin sulfate which is expressed by neurons and astrocytes[22] and has been shown to be a potent inhibitor of neurite extension in tissue culture.[23]

Stopping axons by changing their substrate may not be a sufficient signal for activation of the physiological stop pathway. When axons are deprived of a substrate or physically blocked, neurofilaments still accumulate in axon terminals[1,21] and neurofilament synthesis in the cell body remains depressed[14] indicating that the pathway has not been activated by the mere act of stopping axonal extension.

Thus, some other signal may be needed to turn off the neuronal growth response. Soluble factors, released by target cells are taken up by axonal endings by receptor-mediated endocytosis and retrogradely transported to the neuronal soma[24,25] where they regulate gene expression.[26,27] NGF is the best known of these soluble factors and has been shown to regulate substance P precursor molecule mRNA levels *in vitro*[26] as well as dorsal root ganglion substance P synthesis.[4] Moreover, NGF has been shown to regulate neurofilament synthesis *in vitro*[28,29] as well as neurofilament synthesis in a subpopulation of dorsal root ganglion neurons.[30] However, since NGF only affects a subpopulation of adult dorsal root ganglion neurons, other, as yet unidentified growth factors may be involved in activation of the physiological stop pathway.

CLINICAL SIGNIFICANCE OF THE STOP PATHWAY

Activation of the physiological stop pathway then, either by normal targets or by astrocytes at the DRTZ may be a two-step process involving, first, an inhibition of growth cone motility by membrane-membrane interactions followed by receptor-mediated uptake of soluble, secreted factors which are retrogradely transported to the cell body where they regulate gene expression.

Understanding the physiological stop pathway is important to understanding axon-target interactions during normal nervous system development as well as during successful axonal regeneration. Moreover, understanding the exploitation of the pathway by CNS glia might lead to interventions that could promote CNS regeneration in adult mammals.

REFERENCES

1. F.J. Liuzzi and R.J. Lasek, Astrocytes block axonal regeneration by activating the physiological stop pathway, Science. 237:642-45 (1987).
2. J.B. Le Beau, this volume.
3. B. Grafstein and I.G. McQuarrie, Role of the nerve cell body in axonal regeneration. *in:* "Neuronal Plasticity", C.W. Cotman (ed) Raven Press, New York pp.155-95 (1978).
4. J. Wong and M.M. Oblinger MM, NGF rescues substance P expression but not neurofilament or tubulin gene expression in axotomized sensory neurons, J Neurosci. 11:543-52 (1991).
5. P.N. Hoffman, J.W. Griffin, and D.L. Price, Control of axonal caliber by neurofilament transport, J Cell Biol. 99:705-14 (1984)
6. P.N. Hoffman, G.W. Thompson, J.W. Griffin, and D.L. Price, Changes in neurofilament transport coincide temporally with alteration in the caliber of axons in regenerating motor fiber, J Cell Biol. 101:1332-40 (1985).
7. P.N. Hoffman, D.W. Cleveland, J.W. Griffin, P.W. Landes, N.J. Cowan, and D.L. Price, Neurofilament gene expression: A major determinant of axonal caliber, Proc Natl Acad Sci USA. 84:3472-76 (1987).
8. M.M. Oblinger and R.J. Lasek, Axotomy-induced alterations in the synthesis and transport of neurofilaments and microtubules in dorsal root ganglion cells, J Neurosci. 8:1747-58 (1988).
9. S.G. Greenberg and R.J. Lasek, Neurofilament protein synthesis in DRG neurons decreases more after peripheral axotomy than after central axotomy, J Neurosci. 8:1739-46 (1988).
10. P.C. Letourneau, Interactions of growing axons with fibronectin and laminin, *in:* "The Current Status of Peripheral Nerve Regeneration", T. Gordon, R.B. Stein, and P.A. Smith (eds), Alan R. Liss, Inc., New York, pp. 99-110 (1988).
11. R. Heumann, S. Korschung, C. Bandtlow, and H. Thoenen, Changes of nerve growth factor synthesis in non-neuronal cells in response to sciatic nerve transection, J Cell Biol. 104:1623-31 (1987).
12. P.J. Reier and J.D. Houle, The glial scar: Its bearing on axonal elongation and transplantation approaches to CNS repair, *in:* "Functional Recovery in Neurological Diseases. Advances in Neurology", v. 47 S.G. Waxman (ed), Raven Press, New York, pp.87-138 (1988).
13. F.J. Liuzzi, Proteolysis is a critical step in the physiological stop pathway: mechanisms involved in the blockade of axonal regeneration by mammalian astrocytes, Brain Res 512:277-83 (1990a).
14. F.J. Liuzzi and B. Tedeschi, The effects of physiological stop pathway activation at the dorsal root transitional zone on NF gene expression in DRG neuron, Soc Neurosci Abst 15:707 (1990).
15. F.J. Liuzzi, Regulation of axonal growth through the dorsal root transitional zone in adult mammals. *in:* Advances in Neural Regeneration Research", v. 60, Seil, F.J. (ed), Wiley-Liss, New York, pp.225-36 (1990b).
16. B.I. Roots, Neurofilament accumulation induced in synapses by leupeptin, Science 221:971-72 (1983).
17. F. Liuzzi and B. Tedeschi, in preparation.
18. D. Bozyczko and A.F. Horwitz AF (1986) The participation of a putative cell surface receptor for laminin and fibronectin in peripheral neurite extension. J Neurosci 6:1241-1251
19. B. Toyota, S. Carbonetto, and S. David, A dual laminin/collagen receptor acts in peripheral nerve regeneration, Proc Natl Acad Sci USA 87:1319-22 (1990).
20. A. Bignami, N.H. Chi and D. Dahl, Regenerating dorsal roots and the nerve entry zone: An immunofluorescence study with neurofilament and laminin antisera, Exp Neurol 85:426-436 (1984).
21. F.J. Liuzzi, unpublished observations..
22. D.A. Aquino, R.U. Margolis, and R.K. Margolis, Immunocytochemical localization of a chondroitin sulfate proteoglycan in nervous tissue. Adult brain, retina and peripheral nerve, J Cell Biol 99:1117-1129 (1984).
23. D.M. Snow, V. Lemmon, D.A. Carrino, A.I. Caplan, and J. Silver, Sulfated proteoglycans in astroglial barriers inhibit neurite outgrowth *in vitro*, Exp Neurol 109:111-30 (1990).
24. I.A. Hendry, K. Stockkel, H. Thoenen, and L.L. Iverson, Retrograde axonal transport of nerve growth factor, Brain Res 68:103-21 (1974).
25. E.M. Johnson, M. Taniuchi, H.B. Clark, J.E. Springer, S. Koh, M.W. Tayrien, and R. Loy, Demonstration of retrograde transport of nerve growth factor receptor in the peripheral an central nervous system, J Neurosci 7:923-29 (1987).
26. R.M. Lindsay and A.J. Hamar, Nerve growth factor regulates expression of neuropeptide genes in adult sensory neurons, Nature 337:362-64 (1989).

27. J. Wong and M.M. Oblinger MM, A comparison of peripheral and central axotomy effects on neurofilament and tubulin gene expression in rat dorsal root ganglion neurons, J Neurosci 10:2215-22 (1990).

28. V. Lee, J.Q. Trajanowski, and W.W. Schleapfer, Induction of neurofilament triplet in PC12 cells by nerve growth factor, Brain Res 238:169-80 (1982).

29. M.H. Lindenbaum, S. Carbonetto, and W.E. Mushyski, Nerve growth factor enhances the synthesis, phosphorylation, and metabolic stability of neurofilament proteins in PC12 cells, J Biological Chem 262:605-10 (1987).

30. V.M.K. Verge, W. Tetzlaff, M.A. Bisby, and P.M. Richardson, Influence of nerve growth factor on neurofilament gene expression in mature primary sensory neurons, J Neurosci 10:2018-25 (1990).

CALCIUM REGULATION OF MYOSIN I -

A MOTOR FOR MEMBRANE MOVEMENT

Jimmy H. Collins, Ph.D.,[1] Helena Swanljung-Collins, Ph.D.[1]

[1]Eastern Virginia Medical School
Department of Biochemistry
Norfolk VA, 23401

INTRODUCTION

Calcium (Ca^{2+}) is essential as a second messenger in the activation of a variety of cell processes including mechanoenzyme function, structural changes and regulation of exocrine and endocrine secretions. Ca^{2+} may regulate cellular processes as a necessary ion for the association of calmodulin with some target protein. Conversely, Ca^{2+} induces the dissociation of calmodulin from other proteins, including neuromodulin and brush border myocin I. Ca^{2+} also participates in the phosphoinositide cascade, wherein the hydrolysis of phosphoinositol bisphosphate yields a diacylglycerol that activates protein kinase C (PKC) (in the presence of phospholipids such as phosphatidylserine) and phosphorylates proteins participating in mechanoenzyme function. A prototype for the study of the role of Ca^{2+} in these cellular mechanisms is the more contractile protein myosin I.

Brush border myosin I (BBMI) from chicken intestine is the most extensively characterized example in vertebrates of the recently discovered myosin I-type enzymes found in a variety of eukaryotic organisms.[1-4] Evidence from *in vitro* motility assays and biochemical, genetic and immunological studies suggests that these monomeric myosins, including BBMI,[5-8] are membrane-bound motors that can move the membrane along actin filaments.[9] In the brush border, myosin I is present as a helical array of cross-bridges between the plasma membrane and the actin filament bundle in microvilli, and is also associated with the rootlets of these bundles and with small vesicles in the terminal web of vertebrate intestinal epithelial cells. The physiological roles of myosin I in the brush border have not yet been determined, but may be related to myosin I-based movements in other cells believed to include, for example, the formation of pseudopods and filopodia, endocytosis, exocytosis and transport of organelles.[1,10-11] It has been proposed that BBMI may transport vesicles along microvillar actin rootlets in the terminal web to the base of the microvilli and then attach the membrane to the microvillar actin core as the vesicles fuse into the elongating microvilli.[12]

Brush border and other myosins I contain a single heavy chain with a globular head domain of $\approx$ 80 kDa containing the ATPase catalytic site and ATP-sensitive actin binding site. They lack a coiled-coil, alpha-helical tail, characteristic of myosins II and, instead, have COOH-terminal tails with diverse primary structures. The tails contain a highly positively charged region believed to be involved in the largely electrostatic binding to anionic phospholipids.[13-15] BBMI is unique among both myosins I and II in having CaM, the ubiquitous Ca^{2+} receptor,[16] as its light chains.[8,17] In contrast to many Ca^{2+}- dependent CaM-binding proteins, the CaM protein is bound in the absence of Ca^{2+}.[8,17-18] A CaM-binding region has been identified in the head-neck portion of the BBMI heavy chain.[13,17-21]

Ca^{2+} and CaM have been shown to regulate the structure and mechanoenzyme functions of BBMI *in vitro*.[5-8,17,21-22] We recently showed that whether Ca^{2+} stimulates or inhibits the actin-activated Mg^{2+}-ATPase and contractile activity of non-membrane bound BBMI, is determined by the extent of the highly temperature-dependent, Ca^{2+}-induced, dissociation of CaM from the enzyme.[8] We describe here three events that we have recently found to be regulated by Ca^{2+}. Phosphorylation of BBMI by protein kinase C, the association of BBMI with phosphatidylserine (PS) and the association of CaM with BBMI, are regulated by Ca^{2+}. These findings suggest that BBMI is an excellent model for studying the role of Ca^{2+} in cellular processes. Ca^{2+} appears to weaken the bond of BBMI in calmodulin facilitating binding of phosphatidylserine. This binding promotes phosphorylation of BBMI by PKC which may be the initial step in BBMI activation.

RESULTS

Phosphorylation of BBMI Is Regulated by Ca^{2+}

PKC is believed to have a role in regulating many cell events.[23-24] It is present in the cytoplasm and brush borders of intestinal epithelial cells,[25] and has been implicated in cell differentiation,[26] electrolyte transport,[27-28] and vitamin D-induced transepithelial Ca^{2+} transport.[29] We have found for the first time that BBMI is phosphorylated by PKC, isolated for these studies from chicken intestinal epithelial cells. Phosphorylation of BBMI occurs only on the heavy chain and not on the CaM light chains. Phosphoaminoacid analysis shows that both serine and threonine are phosphorylated and peptide mapping studies show that the sites are within about 20 kDa of the COOH-terminus of the heavy chain. The number and location of the phosphorylation sites have not been established, and will require sequencing studies that are in progress. The effects of phosphorylation on the functions of BBMI also need to be established.

Phosphorylation of BBMI by PKC is Ca^{2+}- and PS-dependent and is stimulated 8-10-fold by diacylglycerol. This activator can be generated *in vivo* in response to receptor-mediated activation of the phosphoinositide signaling pathway.[23-24] The effects of Ca^{2+} on the phosphorylation of BBMI by PKC were studied in greater detail by determining the amount of phosphate incorporated into BBMI in the initial phase of the reaction in the presence of PKC, PS and DOG at Ca^{2+} concentrations from < 10^{-8} M to 320 μM (Fig 1A). A peak in phosphorylation occurred at 3 μM Ca^{2+}. At Ca^{2+} concentrations from < 10^{-8} m to 0.5 μM, phosphorylation was essentially constant at ≈ 25% of the maximal level. Stimulation occurred in the narrow range of 0.5 to 3 μM Ca^{2+}, with 1.3 μM Ca^{2+} producing half-maximal stimulation. At Ca^{2+} levels > 3 μM Ca^{2+}, BBMI phosphorylation decreased, with a decline in phosphorylation of nearly 60% occurring between 3 and 13 μM Ca^{2+}. The effects of Ca^{2+} on BBMI phosphorylation are clearly more complex than has been found for phosphorylation of histones by PKC,[30] including the enzyme from intestinal epithelial cells.[25] For histones, increasing the Ca^{2+} concentration from ≈ 0.1 to 1 μM stimulates phosphorylation, and inhibition has not been observed at higher Ca^{2+} levels. This effect may be central to the nature of the function of the motility protein.

Ca^{2+} Regulates BBMI Phosphorylation by PKC by Stimulating the Binding of BBMI to Phosphatidylserine.

To attempt to understand the mechanism of regulation of PKC phosphorylation of BBMI by Ca^{2+}, we studied the effects of Ca^{2+} on the binding of BBMI to the PS vesicles present in the kinase assay mixtures. For studies of BBMI binding to PS vesicles, BBMI was co-sedimented with PS vesicles present in phosphorylation mixtures at Ca^{2+} concentrations from < 10 μM to 320 μM at 100,000 x g for 60 min. The distribution of BBMI between supernatant and pellet fractions was determined by SDS-PAGE and

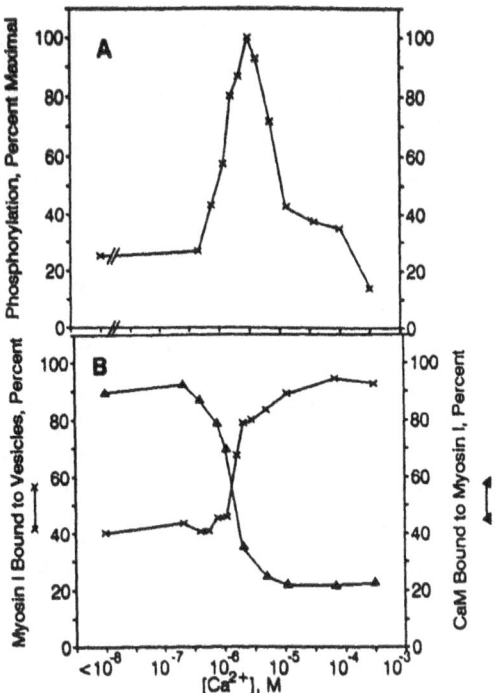

Figure 1. Effects of Ca^{2+} on phosphorylation of BBMI by PKC, binding of BBMI to PS vesicles and dissociation of CaM from BBMI. *Panel A*, BBMI was incubated with PKC in the presence of PS, diacylglycerol and $CaCl_2$ to give the indicated free Ca^{2+} concentrations for 2 min at 30° C and aliquots were analyzed by SDS-PAGE and autoradiography. ^{32}P incorporation was determined on heavy chains excised from the gel and expressed as a percentage of the maximal incorporation (0.28 mol P/mol heavy chain). The values shown are the averages of five experiments. *Panel B*, (x--x) shows the binding of BBMI to PS vesicles. BBMI was incubated with PKC in the presence of PS, diacylglycerol and the indicated free Ca^{2+} concentrations for 2 min at 30° C. The samples were centrifuged at 100,000 x g for 60 min and equal aliquots of the supernatant and pellet fractions were analyzed by SDS-PAGE. The distribution of BBMI heavy chain in the fractions was determined by densitometry of the gel and expressed as a percentage of BBMI bound to vesicles in the pellet. *Panel B*, (Δ--Δ): BBMI was incubated as above except that rabbit skeletal muscle F-actin was present. After 2 min, hexokinase and D-glucose were added and the incubation was continued for 20 min at 23 °C to deplete ATP present in the incubation mixtures. The samples were then centrifuged at 100,000 x g for 20 min and supernatant and pellet fractions were analyzed by SDS-PAGE. The distribution of CaM in the fractions was determined by densitometry of the gel and expressed as a percentage of CaM dissociated from BBMI.

densitometry (Figure 1B). Approximately 40% of the BBMI co-sedimented with vesicles at Ca^{2+} concentrations ≤ 1 μM. Binding sharply increased to about 80% at ≈ 2 μM Ca^{2+}, then plateaued at 94% at ≈ 35 μM Ca^{2+}. The Ca^{2+} concentration required for half-maximal stimulation of binding was 1.6 μM.

BBMI binding to PS vesicles is stimulated over the same narrow range of Ca^{2+} concentrations that stimulate phosphorylation, with half-maximal stimulation occurring at almost identical Ca^{2+} concentrations. The results show that BBMI is phosphorylated only when bound to vesicles. At both pCa 6.4 and 5.3, only BBMI heavy chain in the pellet fraction was phosphorylated. We therefore conclude that Ca^{2+} stimulation of phosphorylation is at least partly due to a Ca^{2+}-induced increase in BBMI bound to vesicles.

Ca^{2+} Dissociates Calmodulin from BBMI in the Presence of Phosphatidylserine

In the vesicle binding experiments described in the previous section, significant amounts of CaM apparently dissociated from BBMI, especially at Ca^{2+} concentrations > 1 μM. This was qualitatively indicated by the SDS-PAGE patterns that showed a disproportionately high amount of CaM, compared to BBMI heavy chain, in the supernatant fractions. Some CaM dissociation was also observed in the absence of Ca^{2+} in the phospholipid binding studies of Hayden et al.[13] To determine the extent of the dissociation, it was necessary to repeat the experiments with actin added to the incubation mixtures to achieve quantitative sedimentation of BBMI, after depletion of ATP. The distribution between dissociated CaM in the supernatant fractions and CaM bound to BBMI in the pellet fractions was then determined by SDS-PAGE and densitometry. The results in Figure 1B show that about 10% of the CaM is dissociated from BBMI'at Ca^{2+} concentrations below ≈ 0.4 μM. Increasing the Ca^{2+} concentration to 5 μM results in the dissociation of 78%, or about three of the four CaMs. The largest increase in CaM dissociation occurred between 0.4 - 5.0 μM Ca^{2+}, with a value of 1.4 μM for the concentration of Ca^{2+} required for half-maximal stimulation of dissociation. These Ca^{2+} requirements are very similar to those for phosphorylation and vesicle binding. The dissociation of CaM is not due to Ca^{2+} alone, since at 30° C BBMI retains its four CaMs at Ca^{2+} concentrations up to 25 μM, and only one CaM dissociates at > 25 μM Ca^{2+}.[8] Therefore, the dissociation of about 10% of the CaM observed here at Ca^{2+} < 0.4 μM must be due to interaction of BBMI with PS. More significantly, the dissociation of an additional 68% of the CaM observed at Ca^{2+} concentrations greater than 0.4 and 5.0 μM must be due to the combined effects of Ca^{2+} and PS. The close correspondence in Ca^{2+} requirements for CaM dissociation from BBMI and BBMI binding to vesicles strongly suggests that vesicle binding in the presence of Ca^{2+} induces the CaM dissociation.

CONCLUSIONS

Regulation of cell function occurs by a number of pathways involving Ca^{2+}. Ca^{2+} may participate by facilitating phospholipid catalyzed, protein kinase C-induced phosphorylation of proteins, as well as by disassociating CaM. Chicken intestinal BBMI is shown here to be the first myosin I phosphorylated by PKC and the first mechanoenzyme that binds PS in a Ca^{2+}-stimulated manner. Furthermore, we show that Ca^{2+}-stimulated PS binding and CaM dissociation regulates BBMI phosphorylation by PKC. A likely mechanism of the Ca^{2+}-stimulated PS binding is that Ca^{2+} causes conformational changes in CaM that weaken CaM binding to the heavy chain, thus allowing competitive displacement of CaM by PS. Such a mechanism is consistent with the finding that PS strongly promotes CaM dissociation. The physiological significance of CaM dissociation is not known. However, in the specialized case of the intestinal brush border, possible release of Ca^{2+}-loaded CaM from BBMI might be one of the first steps in the transport of nutritional Ca^{2+} through these cells. Finally, these studies indicate that BBMI may be regulated by both phosphoinositide and Ca^{2+}/CaM signalling pathways. This model provides new insights into the probable cross-talk between the two signalling pathways and establishes new avenues for exploration of the signalling mechanism involved in cell growth and secretion, as well as motion.

REFERENCES

1. T.D. Pollard, S.K. Doberstein, and H.G. Zot, Myosin-I, Annu Rev Physiol. 53:653-81 (1991).
2. M. Mooseker, Organization, chemistry, and assembly of the cytoskeletal apparatus of the intestinal brush border, Ann Rev Cell Biol. 1:209-41 (1985).
3. D. Louvard, The function of the major cytoskeletal components of the brush border, Curr Opin Cell Biol. 1:51-57 (1989).
4. E.D. Korn and J.A.I. Hammer, Myosin I, Curr Opin Cell Biol. 2:57-61 (1990).
5. K. Collins, J.R. Sellers, and P. Matsudaira, Calmodulin dissociation regulates brush border myosin I (110-kD-calmodulin) mechanochemical activity *in vitro*, J Cell Biol. 110:1137-47 (1990).
6. M. Mooseker and T.R. Coleman, J Cell Biol. 108:2395-2400 (1989).
7. M. Mooseker, K.A. Conzelman, T.R. Coleman, J.E. Heuser, and M.P.J. Sheetz, Characterization of intestinal microvillar membrane disks: detergent-resistant membrane sheets enriched in associated brush border myosin I (110K-calmodulin), J Cell Biol. 109:1153-61 (1989).
8. H. Swanljung-Collins and J. H. Collins, Ca2+ stimulates the Mg2(+)-ATPase activity of brush border myosin I with three or four calmodulin light chains but inhibits with less than two bound, J Biol Chem. 266:1312-19 (1991).
9. R.J. Adams and T.D. Pollard, Membrane-bound myosin-I provides new mechanism in cell motility, Cell Motil Cytoskeleton. 14:178-82 (1989).

10. Y. Fukui, T.J. Lynch, H. Brzeska, and E.D. Korn, Myosin I is located at the leading edges of locomoting Dictyosteliia amaoebae, Nature. 341:328-31 (1989).
11. J.A. Spudich, Cell Regul. 1:1-11 (1989).
12. K.R. Fath, S.D. Obenauf, and D.R. Burgess, Cytoskeletal protein and mRNA accumulation during brush border formation in adult chicken enterocytes, Development. 109:449-59 (1990).
13. S.M. Hayden, J.S. Wolenski, and M.S. Mooseker, Binding of brush border myosin I to phospholipid vesicles, J Cell Biol. 111:443-51 (1990).
14. R.J. Adams and T.D. Pollard, Binding of myosin I to membrane lipids, Nature. 340:565-68 (1989).
15. H. Miyata, B. Bowers, and E.D. Korn, Plasma membrane association of Acanthamaoeba myosin I, J Cell Biol. 109:1519-28 (1989).
16. C.B. Klee and T.C. Vanaman, Calmodulin, Adv Protein Chem. 35:213-321 (1982).
17. L.M. Coluccio, and A. Bretscher, Mapping of the microvillar 110K-calmodulin complex: calmodulin-associated or -free fragments of the 110-kD polypeptide bind F-actin and reaction ATPase activity, J Cell Biol. 106:367-73 (1988).
18. J.M. Carboni, K.A. Conzelman, R.A. Adams, D.A. Kaiser, T.D. Pollard, and M.S. Mooseker, Structural and immunological characterization of the myosin-like 110-kD subunit of the intestinal microvillar 110K-calmodulin complex: evidence for discrete myosin head and calmodulin-binding domains, J Cell Biol. 107:1749-57 (1988).
19. M. Hoshimaru, Y. Fujio, K. Sobue, T. Sugimoto, and S. Nakanishi, Immunochemical evidence that myosin I heavy chain-like protein is identical to the 110-kilodalton brush-border protein, J Biochem. 106:455-59 (1989).
20. D.J. Halsall and J.A. Hammer, A second isoform of chicken brush border myosin I contains a 290 residue inserted sequence that binds calmodulin, FEBS Lett. 267:126-30 (1990).
21. L.M. Coluccio and A. Bretscher, Mapping of the microvillar 110K-calmodulin complex (brush border myosin I). Identification of fragments counting the catalytic and F-actin-binding sites and demonstration of a calcium ion dependent conformational change, Biochemistry. 29:11089-94 (1990).
22. K.A. Conzelman and M.S. Mooseker, The 110-kD protein-calmodulin complex of the intestinal microvillus is an actin-activated MgATPase, J Cell Biol. 105:314-24 (1987).
23. K.P. Huang, The mechanism of protein kinase C activation, Trends Neurosci. 12:425-32 (1989).
24. A. Farago and Y. Nishizuka, Protein kinase C in membrane signalling, FEBS Lett. 268:350-54 (1990).
25. G. Velasco, C.F. Iglesias, P. Dominguez, F. Barros, S. Gascon, and P.S. Lazo, Protein kinase C from small intestine epithelial cells, Biochem Biophys Res Comm. 139:875-82 (1986).
26. C. Rochette-Egly, M. Kedinger, and K. Haffen, Modulation of HT-29 human colonic cancer cell differentiation with calmidazolium and 12-0-tetradecanoylphorbol-13-actetate, Cancer Res. 48:6173-82 (1988).
27. M. Donowitz, M.E. Cohen, M. Gould, and G.W.G. Sharp, Elevated intracellular Ca^{2+} acts through protein kinase C to regulate rabbit ileal NaCl absorption. Evidence for sequential control by Ca^{2+}/calmodulin and protein kinase C, J Clin Invest. 83:1953-62 (1989).
28. J.D. Fondacaro and H.L. Shlatz, Evidence for protein kinase C as a regulator of intestinal electrolyte transport, Am J Physiol. 249:G422-26 (1985).
29. A.R. de-Boland and A. Norman, Evidence for involvement of protein kinase C and cyclic adenosine 3', 5' monophosphate-dependent protein kinase in the 1, 25-dihydroxy-D3-mediated rapid stimulation of intestinal calcium transport, (transcaltachia), Endocrinology. 127:39-45 (1990).
30. A. Kishimoto, Y. Takai, T. Mori, U. Kikkawa, and Y. Nishizuka, Activation of calcium and phospholipid-dependent protein kinase by diacylglycerol, its possible relation to phosphatidylinositol turnover, J Biol Chem. 255:2273-76 (1980).

SECTION FOUR

PATHOGENETIC AND THERAPEUTIC RAMIFICATIONS

AMYLIN EXPRESSION IN THE PANCREATIC β-CELL

Kenneth L. Luskey, M.D.[1]

[1]Scios, Inc.
2450 Bayshore Parkway
Mountain View, CA 94043

INTRODUCTION

Amylin, or Islet Amyloid Polypeptide (IAPP), is a 37 amino acid peptide that is secreted from the pancreatic β-cell. It's discovery resulted from the analysis of amyloid deposits that are found in the islets of patients with noninsulin-dependent diabetes mellitus (NIDDM). These extracellular protein deposits have the characteristic Congo Red staining found in amyloid in other organs and were initally noted in the early 1900's. However, due to the insolubility of the islet amyloid and the isolated deposition in the diabetic pancreas the structure of the primary component of the amyloid was not determined until 1986. At that time two groups succeeded in purifying and sequencing the peptide that constituted the majority of the deposit.[1,2] The sequence of the peptide revealed that it was similar, but not identical, to calcitonin gene related peptide (CGRP). The terms, diabetes associated peptide and IAPP, were initially used to refer to the peptide. Later the term amylin was proposed by Leighton and Cooper based on the premise that the peptide had hormone-like activity.[3]

CELLS OF ORIGIN AND PHYSIOLOGY OF AMYLIN

In the rat pancreatic β-cell amylin is derived from a 93 amino acid precursor. The mature peptide is cleaved from the precursor at dibasic residues that flank the peptide.[4] The carboxyl terminus appears to be amidated as well. In humans an 89 amino acid precursor appears to be processed in a similar manner.[5] The processed peptide is stored in secretory granules together with insulin.[6] In addition to the β-cell, immunoreactive amylin can also be found in somatostatin-containing cells of the islet.[7,8] Although the abundance of amylin mRNA in the islet is relatively high (albeit less than 10% of the abundance of insulin), small amounts of amylin mRNA have also been observed outside the pancreas, in the GI tract and the lung.[9] The precise cell types expressing amylin in these tissues has not been identified.

The amylin that is present within secretory granules in the β-cell is secreted in response to stimuli that normally trigger the release of insulin.[10-14] Under a variety of conditions the amount of amylin released from the β-cell has been shown to vary in parallel with the amount of secreted insulin; however, the molar ratio of amylin to insulin that is secreted from the β-cell appears to be approximately 1:100. This ratio does not vary substantially in response to a variety of stimuli, such as glucose, arginine, or sulfonylureas. In addition, physiologic maneuvers such as fasting result in a parallel suppression of both insulin and amylin secretion. Under such conditions parallel changes in amylin and insulin mRNA levels are also observed, indicating that transcription and translation of amylin gene proceed in parallel and therefore does not appear to be post-transcriptional or post-translational modification of the response to nutritional perturbation.

Less information is currently available about the expression and secretion of amylin in insulin-resistant states and noninsulin dependent diabetes. Although amylin levels appear to be increased in insulin resistant patients and animals with genetic defects associated with insulin resistance, it is not clear if the increase is parallel to that of insulin. Some studies have suggested that amylin is increased to a greater extent than insulin in insulin resistant states.[15-17] Despite this confusion it appears that the molar ratio of amylin to insulin in such conditions would only be increased a small amount, perhaps to 2% versus 1%. Clearly additional data needs to be accumulated in this area and the assays used to monitor amylin levels need to be standardized.

PHYSIOLOGIC FUNCTIONS OF AMYLIN

The physiologic function of amylin released from the β-cell is still debated. The homology to CGRP suggests a potential role as a hormone-like factor. CGRP is a potent vasodilator and is felt to function as a neurotransmitter. A variety of studies have been performed to attempt to identify physiologic actions for amylin. Although some effects have been noted there is still some concern about the relevance of these effects as they have generally been observed at concentrations exceeding the circulating concentrations of amylin. The most exciting observation has been made by Cooper and Leighton in which amylin was found to inhibit basal and insulin-stimulated glycogen deposition in the stripped soleus muscle.[3,18] No effect of amylin was observed in adipose tissue. This suggested that amylin could play a role in selectively countering insulin's actions in selected tissues. Such effects might also help explain the insulin resistance observed in noninsulin dependent diabetes in which a defect in nonoxidative glucose metabolism in muscle is one of the most significant defects. The infusion of amylin in rats has been shown to modify insulin sensitivity; however, the infusion rates result in levels of amylin that are much greater than that observed in normal animals.[19] Thus, the contribution of amylin derived from the pancreas to the insulin resistant state is unclear. The amylin-induced insulin resistance may represent a pharmacologic effect of the peptide. Further studies are needed to resolve this issue.

If the effects on carbohydrate metabolism are not physiologically relevant, what might be the true function of this peptide. Unfortunately, although there are many possibilities that could be suggested, at present there is no strong data that supports other functions, but, some tantalizing observations. Amylin infusion results in hypocalcemia. This effect is potentially mediated by interaction with the calcitonin receptor. The hemodynamic effects of the peptide have not been explored in depth. Local functions in the pancreatic islet are possible. Some studies have suggested that amylin can regulate insulin secretion. It is possible that amylin could mediate vascular permeability or blood flow in the islet.

PATHOPHYSIOLOGY OF AMYLIN?
ROLE IN PATHOGENESIS OF DIABETES

The relevance of amylin and amyloid deposition in the islet to NIDDM is also uncertain. The presence of islet amyloid is almost a uniform finding in NIDDM and probably is not seen as frequently in patients that manifest insulin resistance and impaired glucose tolerance. In both cases it might be presumed that increased amylin secretion occurs along with the hyperinsulinemia. What leads to the deposition of amyloid in NIDDM patients which is not found in nondiabetic subjects? The structure of the amylin molecule does not appear to be different as determined by Steiner and his colleagues.[5] Could there be another factor in the islet, related to the progression to diabetes, that stimulates the formation of amyloid deposits in the presence of increased levels of amylin? Factors which impair insulin secretionary of amylin deposition have not been identified; but, it might be postulated that if increased local concentrations of amylin were not present, then amyloid would not be deposited and the patient might not subsequently develop NIDDM.

Clearly, additional work is needed to refine our understanding of amylin in normal physiology and in the development of diabetes. The possibility that amylin modulates insulin action is intriguing; however, additional studies are needed to strengthen this argument. The role that amylin might play in the pathogenesis of noninsulin dependent diabetes is also open. The mechanism responsible for the underlying insulin resistance is not understood and if this could be attributed to amylin, a link would be provided between the islet dysfunction and peripheral tissue resistance to insulin. However, not withstanding, the atttractiveness of this dual hypothetical role for amylin, supporters of its potential importance must take cognizance of the observations that the peptide levels that appear to be needed to observe these effects seem to be greater than levels found to occur early in the course of NIDDM. Therefore, a chapter in the evolution of our understanding the pathophysiology of NIDDM may be closing.

References

1. P. Westermark, C. Wernstedt, E. Wilander, and K. Sletten, A novel peptide in the calcitonin gene related peptide family as an amyloid fibril protein in the endocrine pancreas, Biochem Biophys.Res Commun. 140:827-31, 1986.
2. A. Clark, G.J. Cooper, C.E. Lewis, J.F. Morris, A.C. Willis, K.B. Reid, and R.C. Turner, Islet amyloid formed from diabetes-associated peptide may be pathogenic in type-2 diabetes, Lancet. 2:231-34, 1987.
3. B. Leighton and G.J. Cooper, Pancreatic amylin and calcitonin gene-related peptide cause resistance to insulin in skeletal muscle *in vitro*, Nature 335:632-35, 1988.
4. J.D. Leffert, C.B. Newgard, H. Okamoto, J.L. Milburn, and K.L. Luskey, Rat amylin: cloning and tissue-specific expression in pancreatic islets, Proc Natl Acad Sci USA. 86:3127-30, 1989.
5. T. Sanke, G.I. Bell, C. Sample, A.H. Rubenstein, and D.F. Steiner, An islet amyloid peptide is derived from an 89-amino acid precursor by proteolytic processing, J Biol Chem. 263:17243-46, 1988.
6. A. Lukinius, E. Wilander, G.T. Westermark, U. Engstrom, and P. Westermark, Co-localization of islet amyloid polypeptide and insulin in the β cell secretory granules of the human pancreatic islets, Diabetologia. 32:240-44, 1989.
7. O.D. Madsen, J.J. Nielsen, B. Michelsen, P. Westermark, C. Betsholtz, M. Nishi, and D.F. Steiner, Islet amyloid polypeptide and insulin expression are controlled differently in primary and transformed islet cells, Mol Endo. 5:143-48, 1991.
8. L. Orci, personal communication.
9. G.J. Ferrier, A.M. Pierson, P.M. Jones, S.R. Bloom, S.I. Girgis, and S. Legon, Expression of the rat amylin (IAPP/DAP) gene, J Mol Endocrinol. 3:R1-R4, 1989.
10. A. Ogawa, V. Harris, S.K. McCorkle, R.H. Unger, and K.L. Luskey, Amylin secretion from the rat pancreas and its selective loss after streptozotocin treatment, J Clin Invest. 85:973-76, 1989.
11. H.C. Fehmann, V. Weber, R. Goke, B. Goke, and R. Arnold, Cosecretion of amylin and insulin from isolated rat pancreas, FEBS Lett. 262:279-81, 1990.
12. S.E. Kahn, D.A. D'Alessio, M.W. Schwartz, W.Y. Fujimoto, J.W. Ensinck, G.J. Taborsky, and D. Porte, Evidence of cosecretion of islet amyloid polypeptide and insulin by beta-cells, Diabetes. 39:634-38, 1990.
13. T. Mitsukawa, J. Takemura, J. Asai, M. Nakazato, K. Kangawa, H. Matsuo, and S. Matsukura, Islet amyloid polypeptide response to glucose, insulin, and somatostatin analogue administration, Diabetes. 39:639-42, 1990.
14. T. Alam, L. Chen, A. Ogawa, J.D. Leffert, R.H. Unger, and K.L. Luskey, Coordinate regulation of amylin and insulin expression in response to hypoglycemia and fasting, Diabetes. 41:508-14, 1992.
15. Y. Tokuyama, Z. Kanatsuka, H. Ohsawa, T. Yamaguchi, H. Makino, S. Yoshida, H. Nagase, and S. Inoue, Hypersecretion of islet amyloid polypeptide from pancreatic islets of ventromedial hypothalamic-lesioned rats and obese Zucker rats, Endocrinology. 128:2739-44, 1991.
16. P.C. Butler, J. Chou, W.B. Carter, Y. Wang, B. Bu, D. Chang, J. Chang, and R.A. Rizza, Effects of Meal Ingestion on Plasma Amylin Concentration in NIDDM and Nondiabetic Humans, Diabetes. 39:752-56, 1990.
17. T. Sanke, T. Hanabusa, Y. Nakano, C. Oki, K. Okai, S. Nishimura, M. Kondo, and K. Nanjo, Plasma islet amyloid polypeptide (amylin) levels and their responses to oral glucose in type 2 (non-insulin-dependent) diabetic patients, Diabetologia. 34:129-32, 1991.
18. B. Leighton and E. Foot, The effects of amylin on carbohydrate metabolism in skeletal muscle *in vitro* and *in vivo*, Biochem J. 269:19-23, 1990.
19. S. Frontoni, S.B. Choi, D. Banduch, and L. Rossetti, In vivo insulin resistance induced by amylin primarily through inhibition of insulin-stimulated glycogen synthesis in skeletal muscle, Diabetes. 40:568-73, 1991.

STUDIES OF COMPOSITE GRAFTS OF FETAL PANCREAS (FP)
AND FETAL LIVER (FL) IN THE STREPTOZOTOCIN-INDUCED DIABETIC RAT

Donald C. Dafoe, M.D.,[1,2] Xuegong Wang, M.D.,[1] Lorraine Tafra, M.D.,[1]
Ronald Berezniak, Ph.D.,[1] Ricardo V. Lloyd, M.D., Ph.D.[3]

[2]Stanford University Medical Center
  Department of Transplantation
  Department of Surgery
  Palo Alto, CA 94305

[1]University of Pennsylvania
  Department of Surgery
  Philadelphia, PA

[3]University of Michigan
  Department of Pathology

INTRODUCTION

In the future treatment of diabetes mellitus by transplantation, the use of fetal pancreas (FP) rather than isolated adult pancreatic islets may have several advantages.[2-3] Most importantly, FP has a generative capacity.[41] However, the various factors necessary for engraftment, growth, maturation and function of FP grafts are poorly understood. In the quest for corroboration of findings by Ricordi and colleagues that islets transplanted with hepatocytes promoted hepatocyte survival,[1] our pilot trials suggested that fetal liver (FL) exhibited a salutary effect on FP. Therefore, we investigated engraftment, histology and function of composite FP/FL grafts transplanted to 3 specific sites: intramural small bowel (ISB), renal subscapular (RSC), and intramuscular (IM). In anticipation of allograft studies, trials included cyclosporine treatment of recipients using doses that were islet toxic.

MATERIALS AND METHODS

Animals

Rats were selected based on our extensive experience with this species and streptozotocin-induced diabetes. Also, a large experimental background with islet and FP transplantation in rats has been reported in the immunobiology literature.[5]

Two hundred to 250 gram Lewis rats were obtained from a commercial supply house (Charles River Breeding Laboratories, Inc., Wilmington, MA). Pregnant rats provided fetal pancreata of 17-19 days' gestation. Animal care was rendered through the University Laboratory Animal Resources at the University of Pennsylvania. Rats were housed in wire cages in rooms with controlled light/dark cycles. Rats had free access to standard rat chow and water.

Production of Diabetes and Exogenous Insulin Treatment

Diabetes was produced in recipient rats by the single intravenous injection of streptozotocin (Zanosar, Upjohn Co, Kalamazoo, MI) 80 mg/kg. Before transplantation, the recipients had at least two blood glucose determinations >350 mg/dl in one week. Blood glucose determinations were done by tail bleeding of unanesthetized rats using a Glucometer (Ames Co, Miles Laboratories, Elkhart, IN). To prevent loss of weight and general vigor while awaiting transplantation, diabetic rats received long-acting insulin (protamine zinc insulin, Eli Lilly and Co, Indianapolis, IN) in doses of 2-4 U/day depending on alternate day blood glucose determinations. After transplantation, during the time required for FP growth and maturation, similar doses of insulin were administered as a purported trophic factor necessary for FP development.[6]

Transplantation and Transplant Sites: ISB, RSC and IM

Fetuses were removed from anesthetized pregnant rats by Cesarean section and FP and FL were extirpated. The grafts were immediately placed in cold (5° C) RPMI tissue culture medium. The tissue was minced into 0.5 mm^3 pieces. In composite grafts an equivalent amount of FP (4-6) and FL was transplanted.

The intramural small bowel (ISB) is a new transplant site devised in our laboratory.[3] The surgically created site consisted of an in-continuity length of small bowel configured into a "U" shape with the serosa stripped from the anti-mesenteric side. The grafts were placed in the resulting intramural recess. The more conventional RSC site was used by insertion of the grafts under the kidney capsule through a 1mm incision midway along the convexity of the kidney. The grafts were then maneuvered toward the poles of the kidney. The IM site was established by graft placement in a 4 mm pocket of the thigh muscle bilaterally.

Cyclosporine Treatment

Cyclosporine (Sandimmune, Sandoz Co., East Hanover, NJ), was administered per os 10 mg/kg every other day, in some experiments. The agent was employed in anticipation of allograft studies but also as a known islet toxin.[7]

Definition of Rejection

Recurrent diabetes after islet transplantation was defined as blood glucose > 250 mg/dl on two consecutive daily determinations. Histological confirmation of pancreas rejection was obtained.

Glucose Tolerance Tests

After at least 30 days of normoglycemia, intravenous glucose tolerance tests were administered. A bolus of glucose (0.5 g/kg) was given via the tail vein. Blood glucose determinations were done prior to the glucose challenge and 5, 15, 30, 60 and 120 minutes after glucose. Glucose disappearance coefficients (K values), were calculated as the slope of the linear regression of glucose concentration with time.

Histological Analysis

Specimens were immediately placed in Bouin's solution. After adequate fixation, sections were stained with hematoxylin and eosin. Aldehyde fuchsin staining was used to demonstrate insulin granules and PAS staining for glycogen in hepatocytes.

Statistical Analysis

All data were logged into a Macintosh SE/30 database for statistical analysis by a statistics program (StatWorks, Cricket Software, Inc., Philadelphia, PA). Significant differences between categorical variables were analyzed with the Fisher exact or the Chi square test. Parametric and non-parametric data were analyzed with Student's t and the

Wilcoxon's rank sum test respectively. A p value of <0.05 was considered statistically significant.

RESULTS

Fetal Pancreas Isografts in the Intestinal and Renal Sites

Streptozotocin-induced diabetic Lewis rats were rendered normoglycemic, after approximately 6 weeks, by the transplantation of 4-10 FP isografts in the ISB site. Normoglycemia developed in 19 of 19 recipients over a mean time of 68 ± 45 days. All normoglycemic rats gained weight. Recurrent hyperglycemia (blood glucose >350 mg/dl) occurred in all 10 rats in whom surgical removal of the ISB with associated FP grafts was completed, thereby eliminating the possibility that recovery of native pancreas function from streptozotocin-induced islet injury was responsible for restoration of euglycemia. Gross examination of transplanted FP tissue revealed a 10-20 times increase in graft volume. On light microscopic examination, near-total atrophy of acinar tissue with healthy-appearing islets surrounded by fat was found. There was no islet hypertrophy or hyperplasia evident. Glucose clearance in normoglycemic isograft recipients was normal with a mean K value of -2.07 (K value in normal rats -1.75 mg/dl/min).

Four FP isografts were transplanted in the RSC and ISB sites for comparison. The proportion of recipients that became normoglycemic (blood glucose <250 mg/dl times 30 days without exogenous insulin) was similar: 71% (5/7) of FP recipients transplanted to the RSC and 80% (8/10) of those transplanted to ISB. The time required for cure was shorter for the ISB group, 60 ± 21 versus 66 ± 24 days, but not statistically different. The mean K values of ISB recipients were similar to those in normal rats (-1.9 ± 0.3). In contrast, the K value (1.2 ± 0.8) for the RSC group was significantly impaired (p<0.05).

Table 1. Outcome in Experimental Groups Transplanted with FP or FP/FL Isografts in the Small Bowel and Renal sites

Group	Cyclo[†]	Site	% Normoglycemic	Mean Time to Cure[#]	GTT K Values
normals					-1.75 ± 0.5
FP	-	ISB	100(19/19)	68 ± 45 days	-2.07 ± 0.4
FP/FL	-	ISB	100 (6/6)	26 ± 15§	-1.76 ± 0.4
FP/FS	-	ISB	100 (6/6)§	59 ± 33	-2.06 ± 0.2
FP	+	ISB	0 (0/6)	-	-
FP/FL	+	ISB	75 (6/8)*	21 ± 7	-1.47 ± 0.3
FP/FS	+	ISB	50 (2/4)	71 ± 23	-1.49 ± 0.03
FP	-	RSC	71(5/7)	66 ± 24	-1.05 ± 0.8
FP/FL	-	RSC	40(2/5)	29 ± 11	-1.51 ± 0.5
FP	+	RSC	28(2/7)	52 ± 5	not done
FP/FL	+	RSC	0(0/6)	-	-

† cyclosporine
[#] the interval between transplantation and normoglycemia
* P <0.05 vs. cyclosporine treated FP by Fisher exact test with Yates' correction for small numbers. Statistical comparisons between some groups were limited by small numbers.
§ P < 0.01 vs. FP alone by Student's t test

Composite Fetal Pancreas/Fetal Liver Isografts in the Small Bowel and Renal Subscapular Sites (with and without Cyclosporine)

Four to 6 FP were placed in the ISB site contiguous with 10-12, 1 mm^2, FL fragments in streptozotocin diabetic hosts. A composite graft of FP with minced spleen (FS) was used as a tissue-specific control. The results are shown in Table 1.

All untreated (no cyclosporine) FP alone, FP/FL and FP/FS recipients transplanted in the ISB site were rendered normoglycemic but FP/FL had an accelerated mean time to cure. FS did not confer any advantage regarding the time interval to normoglycemia. Histological examination of FP/FL found healthy appearing islets and hepatocytes. Glucose clearance of all recipient groups was comparable or more rapid than normal controls.

In the RSC site, a smaller proportion of recipients of FP/FL became normoglycemic than recipients of FP alone (40 % vs. 71%). The glucose clearance of recipients of FP alone yielded the worst K value of all the groups studied.

In cyclosporine-treated animals with transplants in the ISB site, none of 6 recipients of FP alone and only 50% (2/4) of FP/FS composite grafts had reversal of diabetes. Seventy-five per cent (6/8) recipients of the composite FP/FL isografts became normoglycemic. (Small numbers limited statistical comparisons between some groups.) Normoglycemia was established in the FP/FL group with a mean time to normoglycemia of only 21 ± 7 days. Glucose clearance after a glucose load was blunted in all of these cyclosporine treated groups.

Fetal Pancreas and Composite Fetal Pancreas/Fetal Liver Isografts in the Intramuscular Site

Sixteen FP were transplanted into the thigh muscle - eight in each thigh. One group received FP isografts with FL fragments and the other group received FP alone. The results are shown in Table 2.

Table 2. Outcome in Experimental Groups Transplanted with FP or FP/FL in the Intramuscular Site

Graft	Site	% Normoglycemic	Mean Time to Cure	K Values
FP	IM	14 (1/7)	31	-2.14†
FP/FL	IM	67 (6/9)*	23 ± 7	-2.37

* P <0.05 by Chi square test
† Denotes successful transplant

A significantly greater proportion FP/FL recipients were rendered normoglycemic than recipients of FP alone (P<0.04, Chi-square). The mean blood glucose in the 6 normoglycemic FP/FL recipients was 177 ± 18 mg/dl in the 50 days following the establishment of normoglycemia. In both groups, normoglycemic recipients of FP alone and composite FP/FL grafts, hyperglycemia recurred upon excision of the graft site. Histological examination of excised FP/FL grafts found numerous well-granulated islets and hepatocytes.

DISCUSSION

Transplantation of FP for treatment of diabetes has many theoretical advantages. Human FP has been shown to mature and function (cure streptozotocin-induced diabetic mice), as well as, undergo selective endocrine differentiation when transplanted into nude mice.[8] FP will remain viable and functional after cryopreservation for 24 hours.[9] Cultured porcine FP allografts transplanted to omental pouches normalized glucose levels in streptozotocin-induced diabetic pigs immunosuppressed with cyclosporine and azathioprine.[10] Results such as these in large animal models suggest that clinical application may be feasible providing ethical issues are addressed.[11]

In the streptozotocin diabetic rat model, we completed studies using FP isografts. Stimulated by a recent report that the addition of islets to syngeneic hepatocyte clusters placed in the RSC site promoted hepatocyte survival,[1] we transplanted composite grafts of FP and FL in the ISB. Serendipitously, we discovered an apparent reciprocal trophic effect of transplanted FL on transplanted FP.[2] We noted a shorter interval between transplantation and normoglycemia in recipients of composite FP/FL isografts suggesting that FL in composite grafts elaborated a factor(s) that promoted engraftment and/or function of co-transplanted FP.

The work described herein tested composite grafts transplanted to 3 sites: the ISB, RSC and IM sites. The lack of benefit in recipients of composite FP/FS grafts made the possibility of non-specific effects from co-transplanted tissue, such as local nutrition or increased neovascularization, less tenable. There were variable results using FP/FL composites in different sites that require explanation. The advantages of FL co-transplantation in the ISB site did not completely hold up in the RSC site. For example, a smaller proportion of recipients of composite FP/FL grafts in the RSC became normoglycemic; only 40 % in the RSC site vs. 100% in the ISB site. The ISB site may have provided a better vascular bed supporting tissue engraftment than the RSC. The portally drained ISB site provided physiological glucose tolerance; whereas glucose tolerance was significantly impaired with the RSC site. (In future studies, the creation of renoportal shunts in recipients of grafts in the RSC site will help to demonstrate the effect of systemic insulin delivery versus portal vein delivery. Total insulin extractions are also necessary to assess the engrafted beta cell mass in different transplant sites.) Regardless of the ISB or RSC transplant site, the time interval to normoglycemia was shorter in the recipients of composite FP/FL grafts than recipients of FP alone. Therefore, although fewer FP/FL recipients became normoglycemic, those that did were normalized in less time. Apparently FL, once engrafted in the RSC, demonstrated a trophic effect on FP.

Overall, as compared to the RSC site, the ISB site may be preferential from an endocrinological viewpoint because of the potential physiological advantage of portal vein drainage and hepatic extraction of insulin. There is also evidence that antigen processing by the liver may promote allograft acceptance.[12-13] In theory, the portally drained ISB site may offer an immunological advantage in allotransplantation. But we found that untreated adult islet allografts placed in the ISB site were rejected with a typical time course of 7 days.[14] However, antigen delivery coupled with a course of immunosuppression may yield a different result.[15]

Cyclosporine toxicity was overcome by composite FP/FL grafts in the ISB. The failure of protection from cyclosporine toxicity by co-transplanted FL in the RSC site may be attributed to known higher local cyclosporine levels in the ISB site.[3] Cyclosporine has been reported to have a hepatotrophic effect.[16] By fostering FL growth, cyclosporine may also have indirectly promoted FP growth. Co-transplanted FL may have stimulated FP islets to proliferate thereby resisting cyclosporine islet toxicity through increased beta cell mass. It is also conceivable that FL metabolizes cyclosporine locally.

The IM site is appealing because of its accessibility and presumed safety. In 1978, Weber et al reported that islets from 35 neonatal syngeneic donors, minced and cultured for 6 days, placed into muscle pockets corrected streptozotocin-induced hyperglycemia in rats.[17] Subsequently, there have been no reports of success using the IM site.[4] We found composite FP/FL grafts were successful and produced physiological glucose tolerance. Success in the IM site may be secondary to better engraftment and/or stimulated growth due to a trophic factor(s) from FL.

SUMMARY

A hepatotrophic effect of pancreatic islets on co-transplanted hepatocytes has been described recently by Ricordi et al.[1] We investigated a possible reciprocal effect of co-transplanted fetal liver (FL) on fetal pancreas (FP) isografted into streptozotocin diabetic rats. FL was co-transplanted with FP in three sites: the new intramural small bowel (ISB) site, the conventional renal subcapsular (RSC) site, and the historically inhospitable intramuscular (IM) site. Overall, as compared to grafts of FP alone, composite FP/FL grafts consistently provided earlier restoration of normoglycemia in streptozotocin diabetic recipients (24 ± 8 vs. 67 ± 43 days P=0.001). The proportion of recipients rendered normoglycemic and the clearance of glucose was site-dependent. For FP and FP/FL recipients respectively, the ISB site resulted in 100% normoglycemia in both groups (19/19 and 6/6), the RSC site resulted in 71% (5/7) and 40% (2/5) and the IM site resulted in 14% (1/7) and 67% (6/9). In normoglycemic recipients, glucose clearance was normal or supraphysiologic except for the RSC site. Composite isografts brought about normoglycemia in 75% (6/8) of recipients treated with β-cell toxic doses of cyclosporine that prevented reversal of diabetes in recipients of FP alone. Co-transplantation of FL benefits FP through paracrine mechanisms mediated by unknown factor(s).

Thus, as compared to grafts of FP alone, composite FP/FL grafts established normoglycemia more rapidly, mitigated cyclosporine toxicity and corrected diabetes when transplanted in the small bowel site. There are several mediators that may be responsible for these paracrine effects between the liver cells and the pancreas. IGF-1 elaborated by FL is the most likely trophic factor. FL is a rich source of IGF-1.[18] IGF-1 treatment of rat islets in culture has been shown by some authors to increase replication, insulin synthesis and secretion,[19] but not by all. Neovascularization - a property advantageous to the "free" non-vascularized graft such as FP - may be induced by IGF-1,[20] although it is not clear that vascularization is necessary for islet differentiation. Other possible mediators of FP trophism include a cytosolic factor from regenerating pancreas described by Rosenberg and Vinik,[21] and Pittenger et al in this volume. Another explanation is that the factor released by FL is not trophic to β-cells but protective against a harmful substance. For example, insulin degrading proteases from muscle have been described.[22] In the IM site, FL may inactivate or antagonize these proteases. Further work is necessary to identify the factor(s) responsible for the beneficial effect of co-transplanted FL on FP.

ACKNOWLEDGEMENTS

These studies were supported by the Diabetes Research Center at the University of Pennsylvania (Grant No. S-P30-DK19525-02 for 1988-90).

REFERENCES

1. C. Ricordi, M.W. Flye, and P.E. Lacy, Renal subcapsular transplantation of clusters of hepatocytes in conjunction with pancreatic islets, Transplantation. 45:1148-51 (1988).
2. L. Tafra, R. Berezniak, and D.C. Dafoe, Beneficial effects of fetal liver tissue in fetal pancreatic transplantation, Surgery. 108:734-41 (1990).
3. D.C. Dafoe, W.R. Smythe, R. Berezniak, L. Tafra, L.M. Shaw, J.E. Tomaszewski, and C.F. Barker, An innovative site for fetal pancreas transplantation in rats - the submucosa of a U loop of small intestinal, Transplantation. 48(5):863-65 (1989).
4. Y.S. Mullen, W.R. Clark, I.G. Molnar, and J. Brown, Complete reversal of experimental diabetes mellitus in rats by a single fetal pancreata, Science. 195:68-70 (1977).
5. D.W.R. Gray and P.J. Morris, Developments in isolated pancreatic islet transplantation, Transplantation. 43(4):321-31 (1987).
6. B.E. Tuch and K.A. Leonard, Insulin is advantageous to the growth of human fetal pancreas after its implantation, Transplant Proc. 21(5):3803 (1989).
7. H.J. Hahn, F. Laube, S. Lucke, I. Kloting, K.D. Kohnert, and R. Warzock, Toxic effects of cyclosporine on the endocrine pancreas of Wistar rats, Transplantation. 41(1):44-47 (1986).
8. B.E. Tuch, A.B.P. Ng, and J.R. Turtle, Histologic differentiation of human fetal pancreatic explants transplanted into nude mice, Diabetes. 33:1180 (1984).
9. D.A. Hullett, J.L. Falany, R.B. Love, W.J. Burlingham, M. Pan, and H.W. Sollinger, Human fetal pancreas - a potential source for transplantation, Transplantation. 43(1):18-22 (1987).
10. Y. Mullen, Y. Taura, A. Ozawa, K. Miyazawa, T. Shiogama, S. Matsuo, M. Nagata, M. Takasugi, H. Klandorf, T. Tsunda, M. Terada, M, Motojimata, and M. Clare-Slazler, Reversal of experimental diabetes in miniature swine by fetal pancreas allografts, Transplant Proc. 21(1):2671-72 (1989).
11. G.J. Annas and S. Elias, The politics of transplantation of human fetal tissue, N Eng J Med. 320:1079 (1989).
12. J. Qian, S. Kokudo, S. Sato, T. Hamaoka, and H. Fujiwara, Tolerance induction of alloreactivity by portal vein inoculation with allogeneic cells following by the injection of cycloposhamide, Transplantation. 43(4):538-43 (1987).
13. J.A. Mattingly and B.H. Waksman, Immunologic suppression after oral administration of antigen, J Immunol. 121:1878-83 (1978).
14. Unpublished data.

15. T. Kamei and Y. Yasunami, Demonstration of donor specific unresponsiveness in rat allografts: importance of transplant site for induction by cyclosporin A and maintenance, Diabetologia. 32:779-85 (1989).

16. Kim, YI, Calne, RY, Nagasue, N. Cyclosporine A stimulates proliferation liver cells after partial hepatectomy in rats. Surg Gynecol Obstet. 166: 317-21 (1988).

17. C.J. Weber, M.A. Hardy, F.X. Pi-Sunyer, E. Zimmerman, and K. Reemtsma, Tissue culture preservation and intramuscular transplantation of pancreatic islets, Surgery. 84(1):166-74 (1978).

18. S. Goldstein, G.J. Sertich, K.R. Levan, and L.S. Phillips, Nutrition and somatodemedin. XIX. Molecular regulation of insulin-like growth factor-1 in streptozotocin-diabetic rats, Mol Endocrinol. 2(11):1093-1100 (1988).

19. I. Swenne, C.H. Heldin, D.J. Hill, and C. Hellerstrom, Effects of platelet-derived growth factor and somatomedin C/insulin-like growth factor on DNA replication of fetal rat islets of Langerhans in tissue culture, Endocrinology. 122:214-18 (1988).

20. H.A. Hansson, D. Edwall, B. Lowenadle, G. Norstedt, S. Paleus, and A. Skottner, Somatomedin C in the pancreas of young and adult normal and obese hyperinsulinemic mice, Cell Tissue Res. 255:467-74 (1989).

21. L. Rosenberg and A.I. Vinik, Induction of Endocrine Cell Differentiation - A new approach to management of diabetes, J Clin Med. 114(1):75283 (1989).

22. W.C. Duckworth, Insulin degradation: mechanisms, products and significance, Endocrine Rev. 9(3):319-45 (1988).

CONTRIBUTORS

Tausif Alam, Ph.D.
Center for Diabetes Research
Gifford Laboratories
Depts. of Biochemistry & Internal Medicine
Univ. of Texas Southwestern Med. Ctr.
Dallas, TX 75235

Giovanna Alevato, M.D.
Hagedorn Research Laboratory
Niels Steenses Vej 6
DK-2820 Gentofte, Denmark

Michael C. Appel, Ph.D.
University of Massachusetts Med. Ctr.
Dept. of Anatomy
Worcester, MA 01605

Ronald Berezniak, Ph.D.
University of Pennsylvania
Dept. of Surgery
Philadelphia, PA

Nils Billestrup, Ph.D.
Hagedorn Research Laboratory
Niels Steenses Vej 6
DK-2820 Gentofte, Denmark

Peter F. Blackmore, Ph.D.
Eastern Virginia Medical School
Dept. of Pharmacology
P.O. Box 1980
Norfolk, VA 23501

Timothy J. Bos
Eastern Virginia Medical School
Dept. of Microbiology & Immunology
P.O. Box 1980
Norfolk, VA 23501

Bartolome Burgera, M.D., Ph.D.
NIH - Diabetes Branch
Molecular & Cellular Physiology Section
Building 10/Room 8S-243
900 Rockville Pike
Bethesda, MD 20205

Ling Chen, M.D.
Center for Diabetes Research
Gifford Laboratories
Depts. of Biochemistry & Internal Medicine
Univ. of Texas Southwestern Med. Ctr.
Dallas, TX 75235

Jimmy H. Collins, Ph.D.
Eastern Virginia Medical School
Dept. of Biochemistry
Norfolk, VA 23501

Donald C. Dafoe, M.D.
Stanford University Medical Center
Depts. of Surgery & Transplantation
MSOB-X318
Stanford, CA 94305

Dangling Gu, M.D.
Scripps Clinic and Research Foundation
Dept. of Neuropharmacology
10666 N. Torrey Pines Rd - BCR-1
La Jolla, CA 92037

Aviad Haramati, Ph.D.
Georgetown University
Department of Physiology
Washington, DC 20007

David J. Hill, Ph.D.
Dept. of Physiology
Lawson Research Institute
St. Joseph's Health Centre
268 Grosvenor Street
London, Ontario, Canada N6A 4V2

Joanna Hogg, Ph.D.
Lawson Research Institute
St. Joseph's Health Centre
268 Grosvenor Street
London, Ontario, Canada N6A 4V2

Takako Itoh
Shionogi Research Laboratories
Shionogi & Co., Ltd.
Osaka 553, Japan

Thomas J. Lauterio
Eastern Virginia Medical School
Depts. of Internal Medicine & Physiology
Norfolk, VA 23501

Jean M. Le Beau, Ph.D.
Eastern Virginia Medical School
The Diabetes Institutes
Norfolk, VA 23510

Derek LeRoith, M.D., Ph.D.
NIH - Diabetes Branch
Molecular & Cellular Physiology Section
Building 10/Room 8S-243
900 Rockville Pike
Bethesda, MD 20205

Francis J. Liuzzi, Ph.D.
Eastern Virginia Medical School
Depts. of Anatomy, Neurobiology
& Neurosurgery
Norfolk, VA 23501

Ricardo V. Lloyd, M.D., Ph.D.
University of Michigan
Dept. of Pathology
Ann Arbor, MI

Kenneth L. Luskey
Scios, Inc.
2450 Bayshore Parkway
Mountain View, CA 94043

Chisato Miyarua, Ph.D.
Center for Diabetes Research
Gifford Laboratories
Depts. of Biochemistry & Internal Medicine
Univ. of Texas Southwestern Med. Ctr.
Dallas, TX 75235

Hikari Miyashita, M.D.
Tohoku University School of Medicine
Dept. of Biochemistry
Sendai 980, Miyagi, Japan

Annette Møldrup, Ph.D.
Hagedorn Research Laboratory
Niels Steenses Vej 6
DK-2820 Gentofte, Denmark

Shigeki Moriizumi, M.D.
Tohoku University School of Medicine
Dept. of Biochemistry
Sendai 980, Miyagi, Japan

Susan Mulroney, Ph.D.
Georgetown University
Department of Physiology
Washington, DC 20007

Christopher B. Newgard, Ph.D.
Center for Diabetes Research
Gifford Laboratories
Depts. of Biochemistry & Internal Medicine
Univ. of Texas Southwestern Med. Ctr.
5323 Harry Hines Blvd.
Dallas, TX 75235

Jens H. Nielsen, Dr. Sc.
Hagedorn Research Laboratory
Niels Steenses Vej 6
DK-2820 Gentofte, Denmark

John O'Niel, B.S.
University of Massachusetts Med. Ctr.
Dept. of Anatomy
Worcester, MA 01605

Hiroshi Okamoto, M.D., Ph.D.
Tohoku University School of Medicine
Dept. of Biochemistry
2-1 Seiryo-machi, Aoba-ku
Sendai 980, Miyagi, Japan

Elisabeth D. Petersen, M. Sc.
Hagedorn Research Laboratory
Niels Steenses Vej 6
DK-2820 Gentofte, Denmark

Gary L. Pittenger, Ph.D.
Eastern Virginia Medical School
The Diabetes Institutes
Norfolk, VA 23510

Ronit Rafaeloff, Ph.D.
Eastern Virginia Medical School
The Diabetes Institutes
Norfolk, VA 23510

Charles T. Roberts, Jr., Ph.D.
NIH - Diabetes Branch
Molecular & Cellular Physiology Section
Building 10/Room 8S-243
900 Rockville Pike
Bethesda, MD 20205

Lawrence Rosenberg, M.D., Ph.D.
Montreal General Hospital
McGill University
Transplantion Services
1650 Cedar
Montreal, Quebec H3G 1A1

Nora E. Sarvetnick, Ph.D.
Scripps Clinic and Research Foundation
Dept. of Neuropharmacology
10666 N. Torrey Pines Rd - BCR-1
La Jolla, CA 92037

Andrea Sestak, B.S.
Center for Diabetes Research
Gifford Laboratories
Depts. of Biochemistry & Internal Medicine
Univ. of Texas Southwestern Med. Ctr.
Dallas, TX 75235

Matthias Stahl, M.D.
Hagedorn Research Laboratory
Niels Steenses Vej 6
DK-2820 Gentofte, Denmark

Helena Swanlung-Collins, Ph.D.
Eastern Virginia Medical School
Dept. of Biochemistry
Norfolk, VA 23501

Lorraine Tafra, M.D.
University of Pennsylvania
Dept. of Surgery
Philadelphia, PA

Bruce Tedeschi
Eastern Virginia Medical School
Dept. of Anatomy & Neurobiology
Norfolk, VA 23501

Hiroshi Teraoka
Shionogi Research Laboratories
Shionogi & Co., Ltd.
Osaka 553, Japan

Roger H. Unger, B.S.
Center for Diabetes Research
Gifford Laboratories
Depts. of Biochemistry & Internal Medicine
Univ. of Texas Southwestern Med. Ctr.
Dallas, TX 75235

Michiaki Unno, M.D.
Tohoku University School of Medicine
Dept. of Biochemistry
Sendai 980, Miyagi, Japan

Aaron I. Vinik
Eastern Virginia Medical School
The Diabetes Institutes
Norfolk, VA 23510

Xuegong Wang, M.D.
University of Pennsylvania
Dept. of Surgery
Philadelphia, PA

William J. Wasilenko, Ph.D.
Eastern Virginia Medical School
Head & Neck Tumor Biology Program
Depts. of Microbiology/Immunology
& Otolaryngology
Head & Neck Surgery
P.O. Box 1980
Norfolk, VA 23510

Takuo Watanabe, M.D., Ph.D.
Tohoku University School of Medicine
Dept. of Biochemistry
Sendai 980, Miyagi, Japan

Haim Werner, Ph.D.
NIH - Diabetes Branch
Molecular & Cellular Physiology Section
Building 10/Room 8S-243
900 Rockville Pike
Bethesda, MD 20205

Hideto Yonekura, Ph.D.
Tohoku University School of Medicine
Dept. of Biochemistry
Sendai 980, Miyagi, Japan

INDEX

Regeneration, 1, 2, 3, 10, 13, 14, 23, 24, 25, 26, 27, 29, 34, 37, 38, 39, 40, 41, 42, 44, 59, 61, 62, 63, 64, 65, 69, 71, 72, 73, 76, 77, 79, 81, 82, 84, 85, 89, 92, 96, 97, 103, 105, 108, 109, 123, 124, 125, 129, 133, 134, 140, 153, 155, 156
Rel, 46, *see Oncogenes*
Remyelination, 37, 40, 43
Renal subscapular, 171, 174, 175, 176
Ribonuclease RNase L, 55
Riboprobe, 114, 135, 137, 138
    antisense insulin riboprobe, 138
    reg riboprobe, 137, 138
Rig, 3
RIN cells, 14
Ros, 148
RPMI tissue culture, 11, 115, 172
RSC site, 172, 173, 174, 175, 176

^{35}S methionine, 33
Saccharomyces cerevisiae strain AH22, 63
Sarcoma virus, 45
Schwann cell, 26, 27, 39, 40, 41, 43, 154
    bands of Büngner, 154
Secretogogues, 92, 118
Serine, 51, 78, 83, 160
    phosphatidylserine, 159, 160, 161
    serine/phenalalanine, 51
Serosa, 172
Sialic acid, 127
Silicone, 37, 38, 39, 40, 42, 44
Sis, 45, 46, 147 *see Oncogenes*
Ski, 46, *see Oncogenes*
Snell dwarf mouse, 14, *see Animal models*
Somatomedin, 2, 14, 19, 21
Somatostatin, 1, 12, 19, 73, 81, 86, 88, 93, 98, 113, 125, 133, 134, 167
Somatotrophs, 14
Sprague-Dawley rat, 38, *see Animal models*
Src, 46, 48, 143, 144, 147, 150, *see Oncogenes*
    c-src, 43, *see Proto-oncogene*
    polyoma middle T/src, 148
    pp60$^{c\text{-}src}$, 42, 43
    src kinase, 147
    v-src, 145, 147, 148, 150
Src tyrosine kinase oncogene, 147, 148
Stem cell, 1, 15, 65, 68
Steroidogenesis, 23, 30
STOP pathway, 153, 154, 155
Streptozotocin (STZ), 10, 13, 33, 61, 62, 67, 85, 99, 103, 113, 171, 172, 173, 174, 175, 176, *see β-cytotoxins*

Sulfolipids, 33
Suppressor genes, 45, 46, 47
    retinoblastoma susceptibility gene p53, 45, 46, 47
    Wilms' tumor gene, 46
Synaptophysin, 1
Syrian golden hamster, 96, *see Animal models*

TATA box, 68
Threonine, 51, 160
Thymidine analog, 87
Thyroidectomy, 29
Tissue regeneration, 27, *see Regeneration*
Transformation, 45, 46, 51, 144, 145, 146, 147, 150, 151
Transgenic, 3, 14, 83, 84, 85, 86, 87, 88, 89, 134, *see Animal models, transgenic mouse*
Tritiated thymidine (^{3}H-TdR), 11, 97, 101, 134
Trophic, 2, 3, 11, 13, 31, 37, 40, 41, 77, 95, 97, 99, 100, 101, 102, 104, 106, 126, 128, 129, 131, 134, 136, 140, 172, 175, 176
Trypsin, 1, 74, 101, 124, 126, 129
Tyrosine, 1, 2, 143, 144, 145, 147, 148
    tyrosine hydroxylase, 1, 46, 93
    tyrosine kinase, 21, 22, 26, 42, 46, 143, 144, 146, 148
    src tyrosine kinase oncogene, 143
    tyrosine phosphate, 149

V-abl, 148, *see Oncogenes*
V-fps, 145, *see Proto-oncogenes*
V-jun, 48, *see Oncogenes*
V-src, 145, 147, 148, 150, *see Proto-oncogenes*
Vascularization, 144, 176
Vasopressin, 29, 30, 145

Wilms' tumor gene, 46, *see Suppressor genes*
Wistar rat, 23, *see Animal models*

Yeast, 45, 48, 62, 63, 114, 135
    Saccharomyces cerevisiae strain AH22, 63

Zucker rat, 10, *see Animal models*

The manufacturer's authorised representative in the EU is Springer
Nature Customer Service Centre GmbH, Europaplatz 3, 69115 Heidelberg,
Germany. If you have any concerns regarding our products, please
contact ProductSafety@springernature.com

Printed and bound by CPI Group (UK) Ltd, Croydon, CR0 4YY
23/04/2026
02095629-0009